ETHNOGRAPHIC RESEARC
MATERNAL AND CHILD H

A unique and innovative resource for conducting ethnographic research in health care settings, *Ethnographic Research in Maternal and Child Health* provides a combination of ethnographic theory and an international selection of empirical case studies.

The book begins with an overview of the origins and development of ethnography as a methodology, discussing underpinning theoretical perspectives, key methods and challenges related to conducting this type of research. The following substantive chapters present and reflect on ethnographic studies conducted in the fields of maternal and child health, neonatal nursing, midwifery and reproductive health.

Designed for academics, postgraduate students and health practitioners within maternal and child health, family health, medical sociology, medical anthropology, medicine, midwifery, neonatal care, paediatrics, social anthropology and public health, the book will also illuminate issues that can help health practitioners to improve service delivery.

Fiona Dykes is Professor of Maternal and Infant Health and Director of the Maternal and Infant Nutrition and Nurture Unit (MAINN), University of Central Lancashire, UK. She is also a Visiting Professor at Dalarna University in Sweden, a Visiting Professor at Chinese University of Hong Kong and an Adjunct Professor at University of Western Sydney, Australia.

Renée Flacking is Associate Professor at the School of Education, Health and Social Studies, Dalarna University, Sweden. She is also a Visiting Fellow at University of Central Lancashire, UK and a Visiting Associate Professor at Chinese University of Hong Kong.

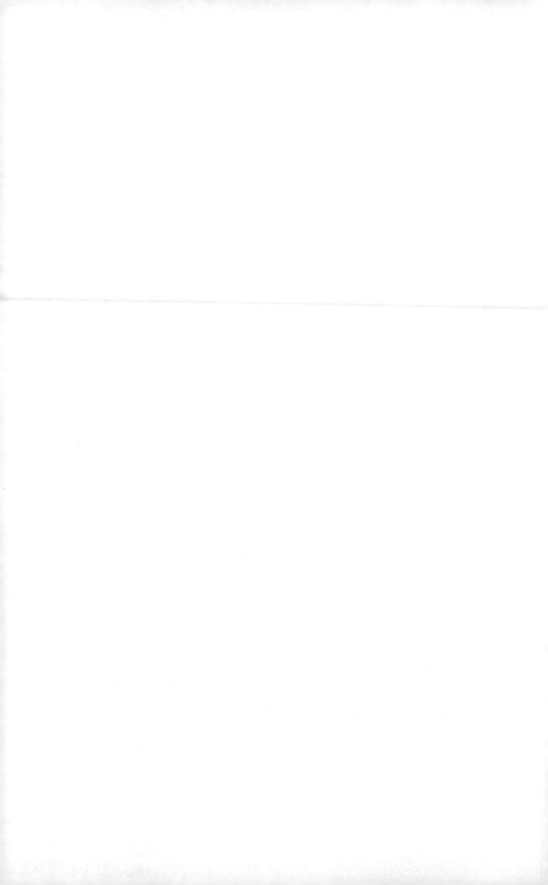

ETHNOGRAPHIC RESEARCH IN MATERNAL AND CHILD HEALTH

Edited by Fiona Dykes and Renée Flacking

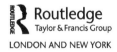

Routledge
Taylor & Francis Group

LONDON AND NEW YORK

First published 2016
by Routledge
2 Park Square, Milton Park, Abingdon, Oxon, OX14 4RN

and by Routledge
711 Third Avenue, New York, NY 10017

Routledge is an imprint of the Taylor & Francis Group, an informa business

British Library Cataloguing-in-Publication Data
A catalogue record for this book is available from the British Library

Library of Congress Cataloging in Publication Data
Ethnographic research in maternal and child health / [edited by] Fiona
Dykes and Renée Flacking.
    p. ; cm.
  Includes bibliographical references and index.
  I. Dykes, Fiona, editor. II. Flacking, Renée, editor.
  [DNLM: 1. Child Welfare – ethnology. 2. Maternal Welfare –
  ethnology. 3. Child Health Services – organization & administration.
  4. Health Services Research – methods. 5. Maternal Health Services –
  organization & administration. WA 310.1]
  RG940
  362.19820089–dc23   2015014491

ISBN: 978-1-138-79220-3 (hbk)
ISBN: 978-1-138-79222-7 (pbk)
ISBN: 978-1-315-76231-9 (ebk)

Typeset in Bembo
by HWA Text and Data Management, London

CONTENTS

ILLUSTRATIONS

Figures

Tables

CONTRIBUTORS

Helen L. Ball is Professor and Head of Anthropology at Durham University, UK where she founded and runs the Parent–Infant Sleep Lab and the Infant Sleep Information Source (ISIS). She has spent 18 years studying infant sleep ecology and night-time care, resulting in over 60 publications. She is closely involved in the development of local, regional, national and international infant safe sleep policies and guidelines. In 2013 she received an award from the Economic and Social Research Council for Outstanding Impact in Society.

Kajsa Brimdyr is Senior Ethnographic Researcher and faculty at Healthy Children Project, a non-profit 501(c)3, NGO, on Cape Cod, MA. She is is an experienced ethnographer who has worked with health care, municipal and technological businesses, using ethnography to understand, appreciate and change the work practice of professions, workflows and services in order to help improve practice. Kajsa is Professor and Advisor for the Maternal Child Health: Lactation Consulting bachelor's degree at Union Institute and University., USA Her current research involves using video ethnography and interaction analysis to change practice in hospital settings to improve continuous skin-to-skin for the first hour after cesarean and vaginal births in Egypt and the United States. She is an author, videographer and executive producer of the best-selling DVDs "Skin to Skin in the First Hour After Birth: Practical Advice for Staff after Vaginal and Cesarean Birth", which is aimed at hospital staff, and the award-winning "The Magical Hour: Holding Your Baby Skin to Skin for the First Hour After Birth," which is aimed at parents.

Elaine Burns is a lecturer in midwifery and Deputy Director of Clinical Education and Higher Degree Research at the University of Western Sydney (UWS), Australia. Elaine has more than 20 years of experience in midwifery and women's health. In her doctoral work Elaine used ethnographic techniques to explore the language and practices of midwives and lactation consultants when interacting with breastfeeding women in the first week after birth. Findings from this doctoral work were rapidly disseminated through six refereed publications, and 23 conference presentations including eight as invited speaker and several invited workshop presentations. Elaine is currently exploring the similarities and differences in communication styles of privately practicing midwives and Australian Breastfeeding Association peer support counsellors. Elaine has co-authored 11 peer-reviewed publications and has a further two currently under review.

Hannah Dahlen is Professor of Midwifery in the School of Nursing and Midwifery at the University of Western Sydney (UWS), Australia. Hannah has had national and international success with grants. Hannah has published more than 100 papers and has given papers at over 100 conferences and seminars with half of these being invited keynote addresses. Hannah has strong international collaborations. She is co-founder of the international research collaboration EPIIC (Epigenetic Impact of Childbirth). In November 2012 she was named in the *Sydney Morning Herald's* list of 100 "people who change our city for the better". She was named as one of the leading "science and knowledge thinkers" for 2012 due to her research and public profile. Hannah has a strong profile in the profession of midwifery. She is a past National President of the Australian College of Midwives and she sits on several peak national and state committees.

Fiona Dykes is Professor of Maternal and Infant Health and Director of the Maternal and Infant Nutrition and Nurture Unit (MAINN), University of Central Lancashire, UK. She is also a Visiting Professor at Dalarna University in Sweden, she is a Visiting Professor at Chinese University of Hong Kong and an Adjunct Professor at University of Western Sydney, Australia. Fiona has a particular interest in the global, socio-cultural and political influences upon infant and young child feeding practices. She is a member of the editorial board for *Maternal and Child Nutrition*, the Wiley-Blackwell published international journal (editorial office in MAINN), and a Fellow of the Higher Education Academy. Fiona is author of over 60 peer-reviewed papers and editor of several books including her monograph, *Breastfeeding in Hospital: Mothers, Midwives and the Production Line* (Routledge, 2006) and co-editor of *Infant and Young Child Feeding: Challenges to Implementing a Global Strategy* (Wiley-Blackwell, 2009).

Renée Flacking is Associate Professor at the School of Education, Health and Social Studies, Dalarna University, Sweden. She is also a Visiting Fellow at University of Central Lancashire, UK and a Visiting Associate Professor at Chinese University of Hong Kong. Renée has a background as a paediatric nurse, having worked in a neonatal intensive care unit for more than 10 years. In

2009–2010 she undertook her post-doctoral studies with Professor Fiona Dykes as her supervisor in Maternal and Infant Nutrition and Nurture Unit (MAINN), University of Central Lancashire, UK, conducting an ethnographic study in neonatal units in Sweden and England, focusing on infant feeding and relationality. Flacking's main research interest is in the area of breastfeeding and parenting in families with preterm infants, focusing on emotional, relational and socio-cultural influences. Flacking is the author of 20 peer-reviewed papers and the author of "Feeding preterm infants in Sweden: challenges to implementing the global strategy in a pro-breastfeeding culture", in: F. Dykes and V. Hall-Moran (eds) *Infant and Young Child Feeding: Challenges to Implementing a Global Strategy* (Wiley-Blackwell, 2009).

Tine M. Gammeltoft is Professor of Anthropology at the Department of Anthropology, University of Copenhagen, Denmark, and a member of the Editorial Advisory Board for the journal *Reproductive Health Matters*. She has more than two decades of ethnographic fieldwork experience in Vietnam and has recently embarked on a new project titled "The Impact of Violence on Reproductive Health in Tanzania and Vietnam" (PAVE). This is an interdisciplinary project conducted in collaboration between the Department of Anthropology (University of Copenhagen), the Department of Public Health (University of Copenhagen), the Department of Clinical Research (University of Southern Denmark), Hanoi Medical University (Vietnam), and Kilimanjaro Christian Medical College (Tanzania). The project is funded by the Danish Ministry of Foreign Affairs. Combining epidemiological and ethnographic methods, the research explores how violence exercised within intimate relations affects women's sexual and reproductive health and the health of newborns. The project places particular emphasis on enhancement of research capacity through a strengthening of interdisciplinary research skills.

Kevin Hugill is a senior educator NICU Education at Hamad Medical Corporation, Qatar. His nursing background is predominantly in neonatal care and he has worked in a number of different neonatal units and higher education institutions in England in a variety of clinical, managerial, educational and combined roles. He has also worked as a member of data monitoring committees and trial steering groups for randomised controlled trials concerning neonatal skin care. His research was concerned with the emotion work of fathers after their baby's admission to a neonatal unit and he has a number of peer-reviewed publications in connection with this research. He is also the author of "The neonatal environment and care of the family", in: M. Meeks, M. Hallsworth and H Yeo (eds) *Yeo's Nursing the Neonate* (2nd edn) (Wiley-Blackwell, 2009), and "Oral feeding the preterm infant: some current challenges and debates", in V. Hall-Moran (ed.) *Maternal and Infant Nutrition and Nurture: Controversies and Challenges.* (2nd edn) (Quay, 2005), and co-author with Merryl Harvey of *Fatherhood in Midwifery and Neonatal Practice* (Quay, 2012).

Mavis Kirkham is part-time Professor of Midwifery at the University of the West of Scotland, Adjunct Professor at Auckland University of Technology, New Zealand and holds honorary professorial positions at Sheffield Hallam University, UK and the University of Technology Sydney., Australia She had the advantage of working as an assistant to a social anthropologist in Zambia before she became a midwife and has retained the outsider view at the back of her mind throughout her career as a midwife clinician and researcher. Now approaching the end of that long career, she is interested in reflecting and writing on midwifery in its wider context.

Daniel Neyland is Professor of Sociology at Goldsmiths, University of London, UK. His research engages issues of governance, accountability and ethics in forms of science, technology and organization. He draws on ideas from ethnomethodology, science and technology studies and his research is ethnographic in orientation. His substantive interests range broadly across: traffic management, waste, airports, biometrics, parking, signposts, malaria and the utility of social science, ideas of equivalence, parasitism, the mundane, market failures, problems and solutions, deleting, value and privacy. These ideas form themselves into a variety of research projects (including FP7 project ADDPRIV and ERC project MISTS) and publications, including books on *Mundane Governance* (with Steve Woolgar, OUP, 2013), *Organizational Ethnography* (Sage, 2009), and *Privacy, Surveillance and Public Trust* (Palgrave Macmillan, 2006).

Colm OBoyle is an assistant professor in Trinity College Dublin, School of Nursing and Midwifery, Ireland. Colm is involved in the education of undergraduate and post-registration midwives as well as the supervision of master's and doctoral students. His doctoral thesis "An ethnography of independent midwifery in Ireland" reveals the dilemmas arising for independent midwives from the tension between the midwifery philosophy of "being with" women, and professional authority. In it, he explores professional authority, particularly within the context of risk discourse around birth and recent Irish and European legislative requirements for clinical indemnification. He has, until very recently, maintained a small home birth caseload. Colm has served on the Irish Domiciliary Births Group and the National Steering Committee on Home Birth, which have nurtured the still-embryonic Irish Health Service Executive's National Home Birth Service. His research interests are home birth midwifery, free birthing and capacity building for community midwifery in Ireland.

Gretel H. Pelto is a Graduate Professor at the Division of Nutritional Sciences, Cornell University, USA, . A medical anthropologist by training, her teaching has focused on maternal and child nutrition, community nutrition, and program planning and policy. During the 1990s she directed behavioral research in the Division of Child Health at the World Health Organization, Geneva, Switzerland. Her field research has centered mainly in Mexico, but she has also been associated with studies in other parts of Latin America, Asia (China, Vietnam, the Philippines, Pakistan) and Africa (Cameroon, South Africa, Ghana, Kenya). The substantive focus of her work is infant and young child feeding and the management of illness in infants and children. The theoretical and policy focus is on the interface between programs (including intervention design and evaluation) and families and communities. She has served on many US and international advisory committees and is currently a member of several editorial boards including *Ecology of Food and Nutrition*, *Maternal and Child Nutrition*, and *Maternal and Child Health*. She is a recipient of a number of awards, including an honorary doctorate from the University of Helsinki, Finland, a Fellow of the American Society for Nutrition, SN, and the Malinowski Award (2007) from the Society for Applied Anthropology given "to an outstanding social scientist in recognition of efforts to understand and serve the needs of the world's societies and who has actively pursued the goal of solving human problems using the concepts and tools of social science."

Virginia Schmied is Professor and Director of Engagement and International in the School of Nursing and Midwifery, University of Western Sydney, Australia and she holds a Visiting Professorship at University of Central Lancashire, UK. She is a registered midwife and a registered nurse with experience in clinical practice, education, research and consultancy. Virginia has worked in other tertiary institutions and as a senior manager in the public sector. She is a leading Australian researcher in midwifery and child and family health. Her program of scholarship, teaching and research is grounded in social science theory and methods and focuses on transition to motherhood, breastfeeding and infant feeding decisions, perinatal mental health, postnatal care and strengthening the universal health services for families and children. Virginia has been successful in competitive grants, has published over 130 refereed journal articles, book chapters and published reports and regularly presents at national and international conferences. Her research has been translated to policy and practice, for example through the development of teaching resources for consumers and health professionals.

Catherine E. Taylor graduated from Durham University, UK and was awarded an ESRC/MRC 1+3 postgraduate studentship to complete a PhD in medical anthropology under the supervision of Professor Helen Ball. Catherine worked as a research assistant on the North East Cot Trial (NECOT) and for her PhD conducted a qualitative follow-up of NECOT involving participants and NHS postnatal ward staff. Her interest is in exploring the bio-social aspects of maternal-infant care with the aim of identifying factors that may facilitate intended breastfeeding outcomes and improve healthcare services.

Kristin P. Tully is a Research Affiliate at the Center for Developmental Science at the University of North Carolina at Chapel Hill, USA. She obtained her

PhD in biological anthropology from Durham University, UK, in 2010. Kristin was a Postdoctoral Fellow through the Carolina Consortium on Human Development through the National Institute of Child Health and Human Development from 2010 to 2013. Her interest is in investigating provider care and parenting decisions in the domains of childbirth and infancy. She aims to contribute to nursing science, advance evolutionary-developmental theory, and improve family wellbeing. Kristin's research disentangles factors underlying perinatal outcomes such as mode of childbirth, breastfeeding rates, and parent–infant sleep practices.

Sera Young has an MA in medical anthropology (University of Amsterdam, the Netherlands) and a PhD in International Nutrition (Cornell University, USA). In 2011 she returned to Cornell as faculty in the Division of Nutritional Sciences after holding faculty and fellowship positions at the University of California-Berkeley, University of California-Davis, and University of California-San Francisco. She has over a decade of ethnographic experience on maternal and child under-nutrition in sub-Saharan Africa. Her areas of emphasis include HIV, nutrition during pregnancy, infant feeding, micronutrient deficiencies, and non-food cravings (pica). Descriptions of her publications, including her recent book, *Craving Earth* (Columbia University Press, 2011) for which she received the Margaret Mead Award, can be found at www.serayoung.org.

FOREWORD AND INTRODUCTION

Mavis Kirkham

This book is to be welcomed because it fills a real gap in the reading available to those working around maternal and child health. Ethnography is a research method which enables insight into the subtleties of the social world, so there is much we can learn from the studies reported here which will enrich our understanding and our practice. We can also learn from how these studies are conducted: habits of observation and questioning which deepen our understanding. Ethnography is not just a research method but an approach to observation, interviewing and analysis which is widely useful.

The skills of ethnography are similar to the skills needed for health care practitioners in maternal and child health. Awareness of cultural context is vital for both practices, highlighting the taken-for-granted and making it possible to explore both explicit and tacit knowledge. Reflexivity is similarly important, requiring us to be aware of the cultural lens through which we see the world, which may be very different from the lens of those we study or those for whom we provide care. Ethnography and health care practice both require the conscious and careful building of trust. Working collaboratively is also important in both contexts and requires a considerable degree of self-awareness.

Ethnographers and health care practitioners cannot identify too closely with the culture in which they work, or they lose their awareness of it. Participant observation is a dynamic practice requiring constant movement on the continuum between observation and participation. Total observation is not possible, except through concealed one-way mirrors; we inevitably influence what we observe and participation without observation would be crass. As health care practitioners and researchers we constantly move on the continuum between observation and participation.

Ethnography is also useful in providing us with an analytical framework with which to view our practice and the influences upon us. As Brigitte Jordan (1993) states, 'whatever the details of a given birthing system – its practitioners tend to see it as the best way, the right way, indeed *the* way to bring a child into the world' (p.4). Yet in our diverse, modern world, such dictates are not enough. Ethnography enables us to identify the origins of 'the right way' in our particular context and to see other ways which may be travelled by those in our care.

The chapters in this book present very different aspects of ethnography and demonstrate the diversity of this approach to research.

In Chapter 1 Fiona Dykes and Renée Flacking provide a clear and helpful introduction to the theory and practice of ethnography. They focus on its origins within anthropology, its theoretical foundations and associated methodologies as well as the practicalities of conducting such research. They highlight the role of participant observer, how meaning is constructed through shared cultural experience and explicit and tacit levels of knowledge. Reflexivity is examined and seen as key to ethnographic research.

In Chapter 2 Tine M. Gammeltoft focuses on 'Ethnographic fieldwork as teamwork', using her work with Vietnamese colleagues researching the routinisation of ultrasound in Vietnamese antenatal care. She demonstrates how colleagues from different backgrounds worked together to produce insights which would not have been open to them as individuals. Issues of power and professional myths and assumptions had to be overcome in the process of 'being ethnographic' and sensitively analysing the experience of Vietnamese mothers undergoing termination of wanted pregnancies because of fetal abnormalities.

In Chapter 3 Kajsa Brimdyr looks at 'Work practice ethnography', using video as well as the more usual ethnographic fieldwork methods in maternity settings as 'a rapid method of making sustainable change'. She takes, as an example, the introduction of the Baby Friendly Hospital Initiative (BFHI) step four, relating to skin-to-skin contact after birth, in two very different settings. This rapid change technique has five steps, a structure very similar to that of BFHI itself. It is a top-down technique for change which starts with the education of staff by external experts, but it has the advantage of enabling staff to watch the videos and see the process of change in their unit. Indeed the creation of that educational opportunity, not available in normal health care practice, enabled them to observe and marvel at the behaviour of the newborn, who was also observed through a series of 'stages' before feeding for the first time. This approach enabled staff to see the problems caused by breaking off skin-to-skin contact before the first feed. This chapter provides a fascinating glimpse of a highly structured technique for bringing about change, which retains 'non-judgemental' and democratic elements in that the staff monitor their efforts to bring about the imposed change with technical help which gives them insight into the change process in their local setting.

In Chapter 4 Colm OBoyle presents an autoethnographic account of how he 'came to disengage from a woman who had planned to have him as her home birth midwife'. This is a personal account where the author interrogates his thoughts and behaviour as research data, and analyses his story in its context. The chapter has three aims, 'one, to tell the story, two, to argue that the story, as an exemplar of autoethnography, can be presented as research, and three, to explore the concept of professionalism within midwifery'. These aims are achieved, though the ethnography here described is very different from that in the rest of the book, as the research is retrospective and the viewpoint that of the one, highly reflective, main actor. Important issues are explored in this chapter which would have been difficult to explore in other ways as not giving care can be discussed but not, by definition, observed.

In Chapter 5 Virginia Schmied, Elaine Burns and Hannah Dahlen use ethnography 'to identify and facilitate best practice in maternity and child health care'. Observational studies enable them to highlight the difference between the rhetoric and the reality of care. They draw on three very different ethnographic studies addressing the implementation of routine psychosocial assessment and depression screening in the perinatal period, facilitators and barriers to physiological birth positioning and the implementation of principles and strategies to support the initiation and establishment of breastfeeding. When studying these different subjects in different settings they were struck by the similarities across the findings, particularly in relation to the approach to practice taken by individual midwives and nurses, as well as the nature of the organisational culture and the structural barriers to evidence-based practice. Using Foucauldian analysis, they synthesise the findings of these studies to reveal the exercise of power: 'the set of tools or bag of tricks … employed to cajole or coerce women into complying with institution norms or practices'. Examples of resistance are also reported where relationships were prioritised and practice adapted to meet clients' needs. As has long been noted, in birth centres and women's homes there was greater likelihood of real partnership between women and professionals. The authors conclude that their work demonstrates the 'futile nature' of attempts to control evidence-based practice from the top-down by setting targets and increasing external control structures to drive through change. Instead they advocate 'taking a bottom-up and top-down approach to practice change and the value of respectful collaboration across professions, services and with consumers'.

In Chapter 6 Renée Flacking and Fiona Dykes present their comparative research in the highly medicalised settings of neonatal intensive care units in England and Sweden. The study focuses on the transition to breastfeeding for premature babies and their mothers prior to their discharge from neonatal intensive care units (NICU). This transition has been seen to be 'not only regulated by a diversity of non-evidence based guidelines and care routines but also turned into a technical process with breastfeeding being seen as a "product" and not part of a relational interplay'. This comparative study therefore sought to examine the influence of differing cultures on mothers' experiences of breastfeeding and the breastfeeding relationship with their preterm baby in NICUs in Sweden and England. Three separate levels of analysis were used: the macro (national/societal), the meso (the local NICU) and the micro (individual's experiences in specific NICUs) and striking differences were found between countries and within units in the same country. This chapter also considers how researchers manage emotions and the importance for them of emotional debriefing. The authors also stress the importance of team involvement to enhance reflexivity and reduce familiarity.

In Chapter 7 Catherine E. Taylor, Kristin H. Tully and Helen L. Ball look at the night-time experiences of mothers, infants, and staff on a postnatal ward. They used 'objective coding of behaviour' collected by video of mother–baby dyads all night in three randomised controlled trials on the effect of the post-natal proximity of mothers and babies on their breastfeeding. This data was examined in the light of interviews with all concerned. Thus they were able to examine actions normally hidden from view by darkness, curtains or sleep, together with the feelings and priorities of all concerned. The resulting themes encompassed the experiences of mother–infant dyads and of staff. It was evident that 'traditional' rooming-in, with infants in stand-alone bassinets adjacent to maternal hospital beds, was unsatisfactory and especially distressing and painful for mothers after caesarean sections. Where the baby was more accessible to the mother by bed-sharing or in a side-car bassinet the experience of all concerned was improved; mothers were less reliant on staff and could respond easily to their baby's cues. 'The stand-alone bassinet was found to be both a physical and emotional barrier between mother and baby.' This arrangement contributed to infant crying, which some staff responded to with formula feeds to enable the mother to rest, rather than helping the mother–infant dyad to rest together. Thus traditional post-natal ward furnishing was seen to cause distress and potential hazard. Together with staff shortage and the cultural assumptions of mothers who did not like to trouble busy midwives and staff who prioritised maternal rest, this very common lay-out of the ward served to undermine breastfeeding and caused stress to all concerned. This is an interesting and informative example of an ethnographic approach to data collected in a large statistical study.

In Chapter 8, Kevin Hugill looks at fathers' emotional experiences in the highly technical setting of a neonatal unit. He draws upon his 'auto/biographically informed ethnographic doctorial study' in order to reflect on some of the realities and practicalities of conducting ethnography in a field where the researcher has worked and is known. Kevin is a neonatal nurse and father of adult children born prematurely and has studied men's emotional management in relation to neonatal care. He conducted interviews and observation in a neonatal unit and the data thus gained was used to create a 'qualitative ethnographic survey' of health professionals. For a neonatal nurse researching in a neonatal unit, the balancing of insider and outsider roles and the consequent expectations of others was challenging and constantly changing. Rather than seeing such balancing as involving crossing borders, Kevin saw nurse researchers as living in the 'debatable land': the considerable disputed area between England and Scotland between the late thirteenth and sixteenth centuries.

In Chapter 9 Sera Young and Gretel H. Pelto use ethnography in a mixed-method approach to monitoring and evaluating policy implementation. They present a wide overview of evaluative ethnography in public health, with a special emphasis on maternal and child nutrition interventions. They define 'evaluative ethnography' as research grounded in ethnographic techniques that is undertaken to inform and improve the translational process from discovery-oriented research to implementation-research. This work calls for strong theory, rigorous focused ethnographic methodologies, and a conceptualisation or framework of study inputs and outputs known as the Program Impact Pathway (PIP). These tools are discussed, drawing on a number of studies. PIP is used to identify the many social and environmental factors that affect the nutrition of a population. A fascinating range of studies in very different settings are drawn upon to examine the many stages in policy implementation and to identify barriers to its effectiveness. They show how the values of local communities, for instance in sharing food supplements rather than giving them to one targeted child, can undermine the implementation of infant nutrition initiatives.

Chapter 10 by Daniel Neyland begins by drawing together a brief history of organisational ethnography, highlighting some of the implications that this history might have for working in health care settings. It then begins to set out some of the themes that the author found most interesting and engaging from the preceding chapters, focusing on what seem to be the most pressing challenges in doing ethnographic work in maternal and child health settings. The chapter concludes with a key insight of the chapters: a move from inter- or multi-disciplinary research to studying collective concerns.

This book shows the great range of ethnographic work around birth, and maternal and child health. It covers traditional ethnographic research which creates knowledge and can range from the study of a sizable community to an examination of one individual in a very specific social context. It can also play very different parts within multi-method applied research around policy implementation. Whatever the focus, ethnography examines how knowledge is socially constructed and used to underpin our actions; it casts light on the taken-for-granted aspects of life. Such illumination can change practice, whether it shows the dangers of normal hospital furniture (Chapter 7), the difference between what we do and what we say (Chapter 5) or why mothers care for all of their family leads them to subvert the intentions of infant nutrition programmes (Chapter 9). The glimpses of so many studies have certainly sent me searching for other work by these authors. I am sure other readers will be so inspired.

Ethnographic understanding can make such a difference for all of us working in maternal and child health and thereby for those in our care. It is particularly important at this time when there is such pressure to standardise practice, often without consideration of very different social contexts. I am therefore delighted to recommend this illuminating book.

Reference

Jordan, B. (1993) *Birth in Four Cultures*. 4th edition. Prospect Heights, IL, Waveland Press.

1

INTRODUCING THE THEORY AND PRACTICE OF ETHNOGRAPHY

Fiona Dykes and Renée Flacking

Introduction

Ethnography is a well-established qualitative research method that involves the researcher being immersed in a community of people and observing people's activities, listening and asking related questions. Ethnography originates from anthropology; it was the methodology utilised for observing and writing about specific remotely-based cultural groups. The studies of Malinowski (1922, 1929) in the Trobriand Islands (now Papua New Guinea) are commonly referred to as ground-breaking anthropological research. The anthropologist would generally spend long periods of time living in the community in a participant observer role, watching and asking questions; making extensive hand-written field notes which would then be collated and written up as an in-depth description of the tribe or situation being studied.

As the twentieth century progressed, sociologists started to utilise ethnographic methods to study local communities and organisations. There has also been an increasing use of ethnography to study health care situations both in community settings and in organisations such as hospitals. Neyland (2008) documents the more recent development of ethnography in the field of management research, although, as he notes, its origins stem from the earlier Hawthorne studies in the 1920s and 1930s in which workplace practices were observed and documented. In this context, Neyland refers to two distinct types of ethnography: ethnography *of* involving academic/scholarly studies of an organisation or ethnography *for an* organisation, i.e. carried out for or on behalf of an organisation.

In this chapter, we focus upon the range of theoretical underpinnings that have influenced ethnography, associated methodological approaches and the practicalities of conducting ethnography.

Theoretical underpinnings

Clearly, the ethnographic approach may vary considerably according to the ethnographer's epistemology, ontology and theoretical perspective. Crotty (1998) provides definitions: epistemology is the "the theory of knowledge [...] a way of understanding and explaining how we know what we know" (p. 3); ontology is the "the study of being [...] concerned with 'what is', with the nature of existence, with the structure of reality" (p. 10). One's theoretical perspective may be described as "the philosophical stance" informing the methodology and thus providing a context for the research process (Crotty 1998, p. 7).

Most ethnographers embrace a constructionist epistemology, in contrast to an objectivist epistemology. Berger and Luckmann (1966) in their classic text *The Social Construction of Reality* focused particularly on "reality" as it is perceived and experienced by "ordinary members of society" in their everyday lives (p. 33). In this way, they argue, meaning is constructed by people as they engage with the world. Crotty (1998) defines constructionism as the:

> View that all knowledge and therefore all meaningful reality as such is contingent upon human practices being constructed in and out of interaction between human beings and their world, and developed and transmitted within an essentially social context [...]. Meaning is not discovered but constructed. (p. 42)

Crotty (1998) makes an important distinction between social constructionism and the rejection within other approaches, to include post-structuralism and postmodernism, of the "existentialist concept of humans as beings-in-the world" (p. 43). In this way, the social constructionist holds on to the notion that "experiences do not constitute a sphere of subjective reality separate from and in contrast to the objective realm of the external world" (p. 45). This closeness to the immediate external world is emphasised by Berger and Luckmann (1966):

> The reality of everyday life is organized around the 'here' of my body and the 'now' of my present. This 'here' and 'now' is the focus of my attention to the reality of everyday life. (p. 36)

Social constructionism, as defined here, differs fundamentally from *constructivism*. Constructivism focuses upon the individual's mind and meaning-making related to phenomena, while the social constructionist perspective relates to the collective shared constructions of meaning and ways of knowing (Crotty 1998). Social constructionism thus emphasises intersubjectivity and the shared experience of culture (Berger and Luckmann 1966, Hammersley and Atkinson 1995, Crotty 1998).

To some extent these differences relate to the degree of relativity embraced. Crotty (1998) describes the social constructionist position as firstly epistemologically relativistic:

> Social constructionism is relativist. What is said about 'the way things are' is really just 'the sense we make of them'. Once this standpoint is embraced, we will obviously hold our understandings much more lightly and tentatively and far less dogmatically, seeing them as historically and culturally effected interpretations [...]. This means that description and narration can no longer be seen as straightforwardly representational of reality. It is not a case of merely mirroring 'what is there'. When we describe something we are in the normal course of events, reporting how something is seen and reacted to, and thereby meaningfully constructed, within a given community or set of communities. When we narrate something [...] the voice of our own culture – its many voices in fact [...] are heard in what we say. (p. 64)

However, social constructionism is at the same time ontologically *realist*, in that it acknowledges that there is a world out there and the way in which we interpret and socially construct meaning provides us with an experience that is indeed a reality for us. Thus social constructionism rejects the epistemologically realist/objectivist notion that "meaning exists in objects independently of any consciousness" (Crotty 1998, p. 10). It also rejects the ontologically relativist/idealist position of constructivism that reality is simply "mind created" (Murphy et al. 1998, p. 66).

This relationship between ontological realism and epistemological relativism provides a balance or middle position that prevents what is referred to as "naive realism" by Hammersley and Atkinson (1995, p. 17). This position asserts that there is a definitive knowledge simply "there" and awaiting discovery independent of interpretation. On the other hand the "middle position" treats with caution the extreme forms of relativism seen in constructivism which emphasise that human reality is simply created by the individual mind or the notions within post-structuralist theory whereby discourse constructs, inscribes and creates.

Culture and enculturation are important concepts in constructionism and are absolutely central to anthropology and ethnography. These concepts are defined by Helman (2007) who states that:

> Culture is a set of guidelines (both explicit and implicit) which individuals inherit as particular members of a society, and which tells them how to *view* the world, how to experience it emotionally, and how to *behave* in it in relation to other people, to supernatural forces or gods, and to the natural environment. It also provides them with a way of transmitting these guidelines to the next generation – by the use of symbols, language,

art and ritual. To some extent, culture can be seen as an inherited 'lens' through which the individual perceives and understands the world that he inhabits, and learns how to live within it. Growing up within any society is a form of *en*culturation, whereby the individual slowly acquires the cultural lens of that society. Without such a shared perception of the world, both the cohesion and continuity of any human group would be impossible. (pp. 2–3)

Spradley (1980) defines culture as "the acquired knowledge people use to interpret experience and generate behaviour" (p. 6). However, as Spradley argues, we should avoid cultural determinism, that is, the notion that individuals are simply programmed by their culture. He argues that culture should be viewed as a "cognitive map" acting as a reference and guide; it should not be seen as constraining the person to adopt only one course of action. Nevertheless, he acknowledges that culture does create in the person a taken-for-granted view of reality and, in this sense, individuals are *somewhat* "culture bound" (Spradley 1980, p. 14). In this way humans are able to exercise agency within their cultural parameters. This balance between enculturation and agency assists in understanding the differences between "tacit knowledge", a knowledge that remains largely outside our immediate awareness, and "explicit knowledge", a form of knowledge that people may communicate about with relative ease (Spradley 1980, p. 7). As Spradley argues, what we see represents "only the thin surface of a deep lake; beneath the surface, hidden from view, lies a vast reservoir of *cultural knowledge*" (p. 6).

Naturalism

Hammersley and Atkinson (1995) chart ethnography's journey from a more descriptive and naturalistic discipline, to diversifying to embrace other theoretical perspectives ranging from interpretivism, critical inquiry and postmodernism. In its naturalistic form, ethnography rejected positivism which had previously dominated in the early twentieth century by emphasising that human behaviour was complex, based on social meanings and continually constructed and reconstructed. The aim of the ethnographer was to enter a relatively unknown (to him/her) community as an outsider and document, in detail, the cultural norms, beliefs, codes of behaviour and social rules. However, the naturalistic approach to ethnography itself came under criticism in that it attempted to understand social phenomena as existing independently of the researcher that could be described and even explained in some literal fashion.

Interpretivism

Interpretivism emerged through the thought of Weber who became concerned with notions of understanding rather than explaining (Weber 1949). Interpretivism stems from the social constructionist epistemology discussed above; it offers a critique of naturalism, seeing it as being aligned to an epistemology of objectivism. The interpretivist view acknowledges that the ethnographer's interpretations are influenced by her/his own culture and the context of the research and thus the findings are inevitably influenced by the researcher's perspective. As Hammersley and Atkinson (1995) argue, once the ethnographer her/himself is seen in any way to be involved in constructing there is incompatibility with the assumptions that underpin naturalistic ethnography.

Critical inquiry

Critical inquiry offers a challenge to both naturalistic and interpretivist perspectives in that it emphasises the influence of power, ideology and control upon the researcher, the researched and uses of the research findings. This perspective is generally associated with the Frankfurt school of critical inquiry and a range of political theorists to include Marx (1970), Gramsci (1971) and Freire (1972). The definition proposed by Kincheloe and McLaren (1994) of a researcher or theorist embracing a critical theory perspective, is useful in illustrating the key tenets of this perspective:

> We are defining a criticalist as a researcher or theorist who attempts to use her or his work as a form of social or cultural criticism and who accepts certain basic assumptions: that all thought is fundamentally mediated by power relations that are social and historically constituted; that facts can never be isolated from the domain of values or removed from some form of ideological inscription; that the relationship between concept and object and between signifier and signified is never stable or fixed and is often mediated by the social relations of capitalist production and consumption; that language is central to the form of subjectivity (conscious and unconscious awareness); that certain groups in any society are privileged over others […] that oppression has many faces. (pp. 139–140)

Ethnography underpinned by a critical perspective is described as critical ethnography. Thomas (1993) describes critical ethnography as a:

> Type of reflection that examines culture, knowledge and action. It expands our horizons for choice and widens our experiential capacity to see, hear and feel. It deepens and sharpens ethical commitments by forcing us to develop and act upon value commitments in the context of political agendas. Critical ethnographers describe, analyse, and open to scrutiny otherwise hidden agendas, power centres, and assumptions that inhibit, repress, and constrain. (p. 3)

These definitions point to the centrality of ideology, power and control in the research process, analysis and theoretical conceptualisations.

Hammersley and Atkinson (1995) emphasise the need for balance between the impact-less ethnography which allows the "world to burn" and the ethnography which is underpinned by a clear political agenda (p. 20). The latter may lead to a filtering out of information, thereby simply corroborating the political point making, with resulting compromise of the data.

Critical medical anthropology

In health care research the critical ethnographer is closely aligned theoretically to the discipline of critical medical anthropology. Csordas (1988) sums up the essence of the critical medical anthropology perspective:

> It takes positions on the medicalisation of everyday life in contemporary society, which it opposes; on biomedicine as a form of power, domination, and social control, which it also opposes; and on mind–body dualism, again in opposition. Its intellectual debts are to Marx, Gramsci, the Frankfurt school of critical theory, phenomenology and political economy. Its agenda includes critique of medicine as an institution, cultural criticism focused on the domain of health, analysis of capitalism in the macro-politics of health care systems and the micro-politics of bodies and persons, addition of historical depth to cultural analysis, and critique of allegedly non-critical medical anthropology. (p. 417)

Singer (1990) summarises the balance between the macro and micro perspective in that it seeks:

> To add the traditional anthropological close-up view of local populations and their lifeways, systems of meaning, motivations for action, points of view, and daily experiences and emotions, to the encompassing holism of the political economy of health approach […]. Macro is concerned with insights from political economy concerning 'what the system is' and micro with 'how the system works' – to include how players act and feel and know, where the contradictions and arenas of social conflict lie, and how power is distributed and exercised. (p. 297)

Lupton (1994), in her critique of illness, disease and the body in western societies, emphasises the importance of combining macro and micro perspectives. She refers to the macro perspective stemming from the political economy approach, emphasising structure over agency when focusing upon the influence of medicine in people's lives. The micro perspective, on the other hand, emphasises construction of meaning and enactment of individual agency within medical settings. Understanding this balance between structure and agency is crucial.

The political economy of health perspective underpinning critical medical anthropology focuses upon the relationships between capitalist modes of production, medical practice, health and illness. These are interpreted in various ways by leading authors in this field (Gough 1979, Frankenberg 1980, Doyal and Pennell 1981, Navarro 1992, Illich 1995). The seminal work of Doyal and Pennell (1981) highlights the overwhelming contradictions between the goals of improving health and the imperatives of capital accumulation inherent within the capitalist mode of production. They also highlight the ways in which particular forms of medical practice have developed within societies that embrace the capitalist mode of production. They argue that medical techniques and technology are the "product of a particular conjunction of social, economic and political forces" (p. 292). Therefore, the existence of any particular medical practice and its associated technology should be understood in relation to the activities of powerful groups within society whose interests are furthered by the development, maintenance and proliferation of such technologies. The medical equipment, pharmaceutical and food industries are among the most powerful. Although the analysis of Doyal and Pennell (1981) took place over three decades ago, it remains alarmingly pertinent and relevant today.

Conducting an ethnography

Ethnography aims to study both explicit and tacit levels of knowledge. To study the latter the ethnographer must "make inferences about what people know by listening carefully to what they say, by observing their behaviour, and by studying artefacts and their use" (Spradley 1980, p. 11). In this way, "the ethnographer observes behaviour but goes beyond it to inquire about the meaning of that behaviour" (p. 7). To achieve this level of understanding of a given culture requires participating in people's lives over a considerable period of time, to include watching what happens, listening to what is said and asking questions (Hammersley and Atkinson, 1995). Thus the primary methods utilised by ethnographers are observation and interview.

Ethical considerations

The ethnographer has a range of complex ethical issues to consider. Spradley (1980) argues that the ethnographer should not simply aim to consider the interests of informants but to actually safeguard their rights, interests and sensitivities (p. 21). Before commencing a study there is generally a requirement to gain approval of the proposal through a university and/or organisational ethics committee which usually requires that carefully worded information and consent forms should be provided to potential participants giving them adequate time to consider whether they are willing to participate. Consent is an on-going process and constant renegotiation is required. At all stages of the research process each participant's autonomy must be protected and maintained, i.e. they can choose to participate fully or partially and without coercion. It should be made clear to each potential participant that s/he has the right to opt out at any stage in the process and the right to refuse to answer any question. Where digital recording is being utilised the participant should be free to choose not to be recorded and should have the right to request erasure of any part of the recording. Confidentiality and anonymity must be assured and maintained at all stages of the process. All typed transcripts and field notes should be anonymised with any names being replaced by pseudonyms. Signed consent forms should be locked away and kept separate from the transcripts and field notes.

Gaining access/gatekeepers

In all ethnographic research in order to gain access the researcher will need to gain the acceptance of specific gatekeepers. Gaining appropriate ethical clearance is a crucial step in this process to include clear procedures for protecting the confidentiality and autonomy of the participants. Prior to entering the field the ethnographer will need to speak to key people who can permit access to the community or organisation; in addition, the ethnographer needs to gain access daily to the site of study. Hammersley and Atkinson (1995) refer to two perceived identities of the researcher, the expert and the critic, which make the gatekeeper(s) uneasy, i.e. "The expectation of critical surveillance" (p. 79). The way in which the ethnographer presents him/herself is a crucial influence on these perceptions.

Observation

Observation enables the ethnographer to become aware of culturally learnt behaviour that may not be articulated at interview because much of the participant's cultural knowledge is tacit (Spradley 1980). Spradley (1980) refers to four levels of participation ranging from "low" engagement to "high" (p. 58). First, "passive participation" involves the ethnographer being present at the scene but without interacting or participating with those s/he is observing, for example standing at a bus stop. "Moderate participation" involves maintaining a balance between participation and observation. This may involve fluctuating between simply observing and participating in some ways. The third level Spradley (1980) refers to is "active participation". This involves doing what the people in the study situation do to gain insight into the cultural codes and rules for behaviour. The final stage involves "complete participation". The researcher is this case tends to already be a member of the group/situation to be studied. These levels are sometimes referred to in relation to the extent to which the ethnographer is an outsider (stranger) or insider in progressive order.

In most cases the ethnographer would aim for a position that might fluctuate between passive participation and moderate participation. The general aim should be to remain in a marginal position, being sufficiently immersed to uncover implicit as well as explicit knowledge but avoiding a high level of familiarity, i.e. becoming an insider, sometimes referred to as feeling "at home" (Hammersley and Atkinson 1995, p. 115). Hammersley and Atkinson (1995) refer to the importance of "impression management", that is the impression given by appearance (p. 83) and the "dual effect" of dress, in that it also has an effect on the researcher. Thus decisions need to be made about the type of clothes to be worn and the general way in which the ethnographer manages her/himself in the field. This links to the level of participation that the researcher decides upon. The researcher needs to be aware of the "Hawthorne effect" or observer effect which relates to the effect of being studied upon those being studied with knowledge of the study possibly influencing behaviour. The participants may become more interested in the subject area or they may change their behaviour simply because someone (a researcher) is showing an interest in them (Parsons 1974).

Spradley (1980) recommends a broad approach to the initial stages of ethnographic observations. This involves conducting "descriptive observations". These are more general observations guided by a nine-dimension framework for informing data collection (Spradley 1980, p. 78):

1   Space: the physical place or places, i.e. ward layout, geography, nursery.
2   Actor: the people involved, i.e. the mothers and midwives.
3   Activity: a set of related acts people do, for example the postnatal examination or specific support with breastfeeding.
4   Object: the physical things that are present.
5   Act: single actions that people do.
6   Event: a set of related activities that people carry out.
7   Time: the sequencing that takes place over time.
8   Goal: the things people are trying to accomplish.
9   Feeling: the emotions felt and expressed.

Once the ethnographic research gets underway, the ethnographer spends more time on "focused observations" (Spradley 1980, p. 128). These involve focusing down to elicit more specific aspects of cultural meaning. Finally, the ethnographer engages in "selective observations" involving a narrowing of the focus further to look for differences among specific cultural categories (Spradley 1980, p. 128); these require careful planning of very specific aspects to be observed. Selective observations are made in response to the development of early theory and the need to test out theorising and assumptions; this enables the ethnographer to build emerging themes. This progressive focusing during data collection is also described by Hammersley and Atkinson (1995) as a gradual shift from describing social events and processes towards developing and testing theories. This includes searching for and focusing upon "cases" or situations which would confirm or refute early theorising.

Interviewing

The ethnographer will commonly ask questions of consenting participants to help him/her to understand what s/he is observing in the field. These may be general questions or specific to certain observations (field conversations). These may be difficult to record digitally requiring taking of field notes. In addition a purposive sample of key informants may be selected with whom to conduct more in-depth interviews. These are commonly semi-structured to elicit specific information about the setting. They may take place somewhere quiet in order to enable the participant to talk freely without interruption. Ethnographic interviewing enables the eliciting of cultural meanings (Spradley 1980) and complements the observations made. As Hammersley and Atkinson (1995) state, the two methods, i.e. observation and interviewing, are mutually enhancing in that what is seen informs what is asked about and what is heard at interview informs what is looked for.

Field notes

A key activity for the ethnographer involves taking field notes of observations, commonly in a daily diary format. The notes may be described as "thick description" (Geertz 1973) and they form part of the analysis.

Analysis

Observational data, digitally recorded interviews and additional field notes are transcribed and some form of thematic analysis applied, for example *thematic networks analysis* developed by Attride-Stirling (2001). This involves the development of basic themes that are then organised into organising themes and finally one or more global themes, see, for example, Dykes (2005, 2006). A grounded theory approach (Glaser and Strauss 1967, Glaser 1998) is utilised by some ethnographers, see for example, Flacking and Dykes (2013). Transcripts are initially coded to identify concepts in the data; these concepts are then grouped together into preliminary codes. During this phase of the coding, each incident is compared with other already identified concepts through observations and interviews (i.e. constant comparative method). Identified codes and their properties and dimensions constitute a continuously developing framework for further observations and interviews. Every incident is coded into as many sub-categories as possible and codes are collapsed into sub-categories and categories, to develop themes within the data and form linkages and relationships between them, ultimately achieving a level of abstraction and interpretation. The ethnographer should endeavour to reach a point of theoretical saturation, i.e. the research should continue until no new codes, sub-categories and categories emerge. There should also be a continuing process of refinement and verification of the codes, sub-categories and categories throughout the research process until there is no further movement between the categories and the relationships between them are well established. This process is referred to by grounded theorists as theoretical saturation (Strauss and Corbin 1990).

As part of the analysis the ethnographer develops theoretical sensitivity (Strauss and Corbin 1990). This relates to the ability of the researcher to become aware of the subtle meaning of the data and involves:

> Having insight, the ability to give meaning to the data, the capacity to understand, and capability to separate the pertinent from that which isn't […]. It is theoretical sensitivity that allows one to develop a theory that is grounded, conceptually dense, and well integrated.
>
> (Strauss and Corbin 1990, p. 42)

Sources of theoretical sensitivity include knowledge of relevant literature, knowledge and previous experiences in the field. Further sources of theoretical sensitivity stem from frequent interaction with the data to develop insight and understanding, asking questions about the data, making comparisons and developing tentative theoretical frameworks, questioning the development of the themes and their interconnections and validating them repeatedly with the data (Strauss and Corbin 1990). Ethnographers may utilise a qualitative software package to assist them in the process of coding data and generating themes.

Reflexivity

Given that most ethnographers accept that they cannot simply be tools for data collection without influencing the field and the findings, reflexivity on their agenda, motivations, experiences and influences on the research field and participants is crucial. In the case of ethnography it is particularly important that the researcher is aware of his/her own cultural "lens" through which s/he sees the world. This is crucial at all stages of the research to include making theoretical interpretations. To assist with reflexivity it is important to keep a diary of reflections throughout the research and it is ideal to have a supportive supervisor, colleague or friend with whom s/he can discuss emotions, interpretations and dilemmas.

Establishing trustworthiness of the research

A key consideration in the conduct and reporting of ethnographic research is the need to maximise the trustworthiness of the research by appropriately representing the area being studied. Lincoln and Guba (1985) state:

> The basic issue in relation to trustworthiness is simple: How can an inquirer persuade his or her audiences (including self) that the findings of an inquiry are worth paying attention to, worth taking account of? What arguments can be mounted, what criteria invoked, what questions asked, that would be persuasive on this issue? (p. 290)

Lincoln and Guba (1985) suggest that trustworthiness may be seen as consisting of four components: 1) *credibility:* the extent to which the findings are credible; 2) *transferability:* the extent to which the findings may be transferred to another context; 3) *dependability:* the extent to which the findings may be repeated if the study is repeated with the same or similar participants in the same or similar context; 4) *confirmability:* the degree to which the findings are determined by the participants and not by the biases, motivations or perspectives of the researcher.

Actions and interpretations throughout the research process need to be guided by the need to maximise the trustworthiness of the research. Close attention needs to be paid at all stages of the research process to ensuring that there is coherence between one's epistemology and ontological position, theoretical perspective, methodology and methods (Crotty 1998). The cyclical and iterative process of concurrent data collection and analysis with progressive focusing and seeking out discrepant (disconfirming) cases assists with maximising the depth of the theoretical process (Spradley 1980, Hammersley and Atkinson 1995). Periods away from the field are valuable in enabling the ethnographer to "step back" and reflect upon the developing analytical themes. This forms part of the endeavour to reach theoretical saturation which, as discussed earlier, is an important aspect in achieving trustworthiness. Throughout the research process a decision/audit trail (Lincoln and Guba 1985) may be made transparent through a peer review and support process.

Conclusion

In this chapter we have focused upon the origins of ethnography, the range of theoretical underpinnings that have influenced ethnography, associated methodological approaches and the practicalities of conducting ethnography. We have endeavoured to highlight the strengths of this approach for gaining rich insights into the ways in which people make meaning of their world and engage in specific activities within the context of their culturally constituted environment. We also highlight the complexities inherent in this methodology and the challenges that the ethnographer may experience before, during and after the ethnographic research. The following chapters illuminate the diverse range of applications of ethnography, some of the methodological challenges and ways in which ethnography can impact health care practices related to maternal and child health.

References

Attride-Stirling, J. (2001) Thematic networks: an analytical tool for qualitative research. *Qualitative Research* 1 (3): 385–405.

Berger, P.L. and Luckmann, T. (1966) *The Social Construction of Reality: A Treatise in the Sociology of Knowledge.* Harmondsworth: Penguin Books.

Crotty, M. (1998) *The Foundations of Social Research: Meaning and Perspective in the Research Process.* London: Sage Publications.

Csordas, T. (1988) The conceptual status of hegemony and critique in medical anthropology. *Medical Anthropology Quarterly* 2 (4): 416–421.

Doyal, L. and Pennell, I. (1981) *The Political Economy of Health.* London: Pluto Press.

Dykes, F. (2005) 'Supply' and 'demand': breastfeeding as labour. *Social Science & Medicine* 60, 2283–2293.

Dykes, F. (2006) *Breastfeeding in Hospital: Midwives, Mothers and the Production Line.* London: Routledge.

Flacking, R. and Dykes, F. (2013) 'Being in a womb' or 'playing musical chairs': the impact of place and space on infant feeding in NICUs. *BMC Pregnancy and Childbirth* 13:179. doi:10.1186/1471-2393-13-179

Frankenberg, R. (1980) Medical anthropology and development: a theoretical perspective. *Social Science and Medicine* 14B: 197–207.

Freire, P. (1972) *Pedagogy of the Oppressed.* Harmondsworth: Penguin.

Geertz, C. (1973) *The Interpretation of Cultures.* New York: Basic Books.

Glaser, B. (1998) *Doing Grounded Theory: Issues and Discussions.* Mill Valley, CA: Sociology Press.

Glaser, B. and Strauss, A. (1967) *The Discovery of Grounded Theory: Strategies for Qualitative Research.* New York: Aldine Publishing.

Gough, I. (1979) *The Political Economy of the Welfare State.* London: Macmillan.

Gramsci, A. (1971) *Selections from Prison Notebooks.* London: Lawrence and Wishart.

Hammersley, M. and Atkinson, P. (1995) *Ethnography: Principles in Practice.* 2nd edition. London: Routledge.

Helman, C. (2007) *Culture, Health and Illness.* Oxford: Oxford University Press.

Illich, I. (1995) *Limits to Medicine: Medical Nemesis – The Expropriation of Health.* 2nd edition. London: Marion Boyars.

Kincheloe, J.L. and McLaren, P.L. (1994) Rethinking critical theory and qualitative research. In: Denzin, N.K. and Lincoln, Y.S. (eds) *Handbook of Qualitative Research* (pp. 138–157). London: Sage Publications.

Lincoln, S.L. and Guba, E.G. (1985) *Naturalistic Inquiry.* London: Sage Publications.

Lupton, D. (1994) *Medicine as Culture: Illness, Disease and the Body in Western Societies.* London: Sage Publications.

Malinowski, B. (1922) *Argonauts of the Western Pacific* London: Routledge and Kegan Paul.

Malinowski, B. (1929) *The Sexual Life of Savages in North-Western Melanesia.* New York: Harcourt Brace and World.

Marx, K. (1970) *A Contribution to the Critique of Political Economy.* Moscow: Progress Publishers.

Murphy, E., Dingwall, R., Greatbatch, D., Parker, S. and Watson, P. (1998) Qualitative research methods in health technology assessment: a review of the literature. *Health Technology Assessment* 2 (16). Available at http://iig.umit.at/efmi/bibliography/murphy.pdf (last accessed August 1 2015).

Navarro, V. (1992) Has socialism failed? An analysis of health indicators under socialism. *International Journal of Health Services* 22 (4): 583–601.

Neyland, D. (2008) *Organizational Ethnography.* London: Sage Publications.

Parsons, H.M. (1974). What happened at Hawthorne? New evidence suggests the Hawthorne effect resulted from operant reinforcement contingencies. *Science* 183 (4128): 922–932.

Singer, M. (1990) Postmodernism and medical anthropology: words of caution. *Medical Anthropology* 12: 289–304.

Spradley, J.P. (1980) *Participant Observation.* New York: Holt, Rinehart & Winston.

Strauss, A. and Corbin, J. (1990) *Basics of Qualitative Research: Grounded Theory Procedures and Techniques.* London: Sage Publications.

Thomas, J. (1993) Doing critical ethnography. *Qualitative Research Methods 26.* London: Sage Publications.

Weber, M. (1949) *The Methodology of the Social Sciences*, Glencoe, IL: Free Press.

2

ETHNOGRAPHIC FIELDWORK AS TEAMWORK

Tine M. Gammeltoft

Introduction

"Honestly, I don't think we can ask these questions," Chi said, shrugging her shoulders. She poured green tea into the cups in front of us, waiting for me to answer. It was a chilly November day, and Chi and I were sitting in the meeting room at Hanoi's Obstetrics and Gynecology Hospital, together with our other research team members, Hạnh, Toàn and Hằng. On this day, we were at the beginning of an ethnographic fieldwork that was to continue for nearly three years, developing the research tools that we planned to use as a first step in exploring the use of ultrasonography at this maternity hospital. For the meeting, I had brought a list of questions that I had developed before arriving in Vietnam. Chi's comment sparked a long discussion. Is it possible and acceptable to ask a pregnant woman hypothetical questions about what she imagines she would do in case an anomaly in her child-to-be were detected? Such questions had been posed in research conducted in the US and Europe, but would they work in Vietnam? We ended up reframing and rephrasing these questions entirely; keeping some of them, but setting them forth in a softer and less direct manner.

In this chapter I aim to draw my readers' attention to the ways in which collaborative teamwork can qualify and enrich the questions and observations – ethnographic as well as analytical – that lie at the heart of ethnographic research. The chapter draws on fieldwork conducted in Hanoi, Vietnam, in 2003–2006 by a research team consisting of one Danish and ten Vietnamese researchers. Looking back at this project a decade later, I reflect on the role that our teamwork played in producing the insights we achieved. Collaboration, I argue, shaped fieldwork situations in consequential ways, allowing for the production of knowledge that might not have been gained if a solitary anthropologist had conducted the research. Anthropological insights are, as the example of our research in Vietnam will show, often produced through collective and collaborative processes, and yet, as Alma Gottlieb notes, "For people whose business it is to be sociable, we anthropologists often have an oddly isolationist view of ourselves" (1995:21).

With this chapter I seek to question this isolationist view by making the collective nature of our fieldwork in Hanoi the object of attention and analysis. Ethnographic research methodology is, as many observers have noted, a question of more than technique. It is a way of being, a mode of "being ethnographic" (Madden 2010). In what follows, I seek to make explicit what exactly "being ethnographic" entailed in our research in Vietnam. In what ways did our teamwork enhance our capacity to capture what was at stake for the people we met? In what ways did we see "collectively" things that we might otherwise have overlooked? I shall attend particularly to two important aspects of ethnographic being: first, the development of concepts and theories, and second, the capacity to grasp emotional experiences and sensitivities. To begin with, a few words about collaboration in ethnographic fieldwork in general and in our project in particular.

Collaboration in ethnographic fieldwork

The discipline of anthropology is, as George Stocking (1983) and others have observed, founded on a methodological myth, one that has haunted the discipline since Bronislaw Malinowski conducted his fieldwork in the Trobriand Islands. The central figure in this myth is the heroic and lonely anthropologist who travels far to explore foreign lands, bravely exposing himself to other life ways and mores, alone among the natives. This myth is highly gendered; at play is, as Gottlieb (1995:22) observes, a "Marlboro Man-like impulse to celebrate individual achievement rather than collective collaboration". Colleagues at my department have designated this macho myth "the Tarzan syndrome", observing that despite its questionable foundations, this narrative and the ethos that sustains it have continuing influence on students and faculty, making some fieldwork sites and circumstances seem more attractive and truly "anthropological" than others.

Given the manner in which much anthropological fieldwork is conducted, the tenacity of this methodological myth is surprising. The history of anthropology abounds with examples of collaborative relations (see for instance Sanjek 1993, Lassiter 2005, Whyte 2014), and contemporary ethnographic research is often carried out as collaborative projects conducted in close consultation with local people (see for instance Kemper and Royce 2002, Field and Fox 2007). Today's ethnographic research is, moreover, often carried out in teams, the data collection being planned and performed, and the material analysed, by groups of individuals rather than by single persons. This is perhaps especially the case in health care research, where interdisciplinary research teams often work together to explore the social, cultural and institutional dynamics of health care systems. Yet in spite of this well-established tradition of collaboration, I contend, insufficient attention has been paid to the concrete ways in which collaboration works in practice and to the ethnographic and analytical potential of such shared work. This chapter is a response to this situation.

The research project on which this chapter is based investigated the routinization of ultrasound scanning in Vietnamese antenatal care and the use of this technology for reproductive selection. Among the research questions that we addressed were these: What value do health professionals and lay people attach to obstetrical ultrasonography as a tool for prenatal screening? How do health providers and prospective parents react when an ultrasound scan detects an anomaly in the fetus? How are lines drawn between children-to-be that are to be selected for life and those that are not? I conducted the research in close collaboration with ten Vietnamese researchers. Six were particularly intensely involved in the research, taking part for the entire period of three years. Three of these researchers, Nguyễn Thị Thúy Hạnh, Đỗ Thanh Toàn and Hoàng Hải Vân, were medical doctors employed at Hanoi Medical University, and three – Trần Minh Hằng, Bùi Kim Chi and Nguyễn Thị Hiệp – were social scientists working at different research institutions. As the principal investigator, I had written the original project proposal and drafted the first research tools. These were, however, broadly formulated documents, and I developed the detailed research design and tools in close collaboration with my Vietnamese co-researchers. During the three years of research, we held bi-monthly seminars, discussing the insights and new questions that the fieldwork generated, and drafting articles for publication in local and international journals. Within the overall frame of the project, each of the Vietnamese researchers pursued independent research interests, taking responsibility for the publication of at least one article in a local academic journal. Toàn, for instance, acted as first author on an article for the *Journal of Medical Research*, focusing on the role of counselling when a fetal problem is detected (Đỗ et al. 2005); Chi wrote an article on family dynamics in reproductive decision-making which was published in the *Journal of Women's Studies* (Bùi 2005); and Hạnh led the writing of an article on the overuse of ultrasounds in Vietnam that was published in *Practical Medicine* (Nguyễn et al. 2005). In the context of publication, we found working as a team was important; as members of local scientific communities, the Vietnamese team members knew of the debates that were going on, and they were in a good position to feed our findings into these debates. Given their academic positions in Vietnam, and given the nature of our collaboration, in short, I see my Vietnamese team members as colleagues rather than as the native research "assistants" with whom anthropologists have traditionally collaborated (Gujar and Gold 1992, Sanjek 1993).

We began the research in the 3D scanning room at Hanoi's Obstetrics and Gynecology Hospital, a major maternity hospital. Although 3D scans, popularly known as "malformation scans" (*siêu âm dị tật*), were considerably more expensive than ordinary 2D scans, many women opted to attain them in the hope of having the normality of their child-to-be confirmed. Every day, one or two research team members were present in the 3D scanning room, talking to women and health care providers and observing ultrasound scans being performed. When a scan detected a fetal anomaly, we invited the pregnant woman to take part in the research. If she agreed, we accompanied her around in the hospital, conducting observations in different locations – in the antenatal care room where counselling was offered, in the delivery ward, or in A4, the hospital's department for reproductive disorders where abortions for fetal anomaly were performed. Our sample consisted of 30 women, our "core cases", of whom 13 carried the pregnancy to term and 17 had it terminated. Most of the pregnancy terminations were performed in the second trimester of the pregnancy (for details, see Gammeltoft 2014). Each of our "core cases" was covered by one of my Vietnamese colleagues in collaboration with me. Sometimes, we visited the woman and her family on numerous occasions; in other cases we paid only one home visit. At the hospital and during home visits, each researcher took detailed field notes, and all interviews were recorded and transcribed in full. Field notes and transcriptions were shared by the entire research team and formed the basis for our research seminars. One of the women was 30-year-old Hồng. Hồng's case illustrates the way in which my Vietnamese colleagues and I collaborated on this research project. In the case of Hồng, I collaborated with Hằng, a social anthropologist. It was Hằng who first met Hồng on the day when she came to Hanoi's Obstetrics and Gynecology Hospital to obtain a 3D ultrasound scan.

Hồng's 3D scan

It is early morning, but the scanning room is already full of people. Dr Nhung and nurse Lan are busy working, and three women are waiting for their turn for a scan. Hồng is sitting on a chair in the corner. Her face looks austere. I walk over to her and introduce myself. She does not seem shy at all, and she is very open. She tells me that she was born in 1974 and got married in 1995. She has had many difficulties in her reproductive life. Although she got married in 1995, she did not become pregnant until 1997. When she was five months pregnant, she suffered a spontaneous abortion. In 1999, she got pregnant again, and miscarried at seven months' gestation. In 2001, she again became pregnant. This time she cared meticulously for her pregnancy and went for many antenatal care visits and ultrasound scans. Eventually, she gave birth to a girl. The child was in a transverse position, so she had to have a C-section. In 2002, Hồng became pregnant again, and after three months she started bleeding and aborted again. I asked her whether she felt worried now that she was again pregnant. She said yes, she was worried that the child might be disabled, as a family in her village had recently had a child with a very large head. At birth, the infant's head was the size of an adult's head. Now the child was around six months old, and Hồng came for the scan today to see if the child she expected had any disabilities. The nurse called out Hồng's name. (…)

The doctor moved the transducer across Hồng's belly. Then she exclaimed: "I see no skull." Hồng looked at the screen, but it seemed as if she understood neither the picture nor Dr Nhung's words. Smiling, she said: "This is my second child." After asking Hồng where she lived and whether she had had any previous scans, Dr Nhung continued the scan, looking carefully at the skull and the face of the fetus. Then she said: "The face is very clear, but there is no skull, no brain." Hearing this, nurse Lan came over, looking at the screen. "How come that the heart beats normally if there is no skull?" she asked. "The heart is normal," Dr Nhung said, "and the fetus lives because of the placenta." Even though everyone was talking about it, it seemed as if Hồng had not yet understood that something was wrong with her fetus. Dr Nhung turned to her and said, "Your fetus is not normal at all. You should go and talk to the doctor in the antenatal care room about this." Hồng looked worried. Dr Nhung continued to take the fetal measurements. "It's moving a lot," she said, "it keeps turning. How many weeks are you pregnant?" "Twenty-one weeks," Hồng said. "At 21 weeks it's not too difficult," said Dr Nhung.

The above is an excerpt from field notes taken by my colleague Hằng on March 29, 2004. As the field notes indicate, the scan found that Hồng's fetus suffered from anencephaly, a condition that is incompatible with life. The day after the scan, Hồng had her pregnancy terminated. One month later, Hằng and I visited Hồng in her home in a village located in Đông Anh, a semi-urban district on the outskirts of Hanoi. We were interested in hearing more about how Hồng and her relatives had come to the decision to terminate the pregnancy and how they had felt about the abortion. Even though Dr Nhung had suggested that an abortion at 21 weeks was not too difficult, Hồng and her relatives might be of another opinion.

On April 26, Hằng called Lâm, one of the taxi drivers who would usually take us when we needed to travel out of central Hanoi. We crossed the Thăng Long bridge, then turned sharply to the right, following a dusty dirt road along the Red River. It was a bright and sunny day, and buffaloes were grazing on patches of grass along the dike. We soon reached Hồng's village. Her house was located close to the village gate, surrounded by a spacious yard with guava trees. When we arrived, Hồng came out to receive us. She put her arm under Hằng's, leading us into the house. As we stepped in, a man and two children got up from one of the large wooden beds in the main room; we had apparently disturbed their midday nap. "This is my husband's brother and his children," Hồng explained, while the three disappeared out into the yard. Hồng told us that this house belonged to her mother-in-law, Bà Túy, and that eight people shared it. Bà Túy had three sons; the eldest lived in another house nearby, while the two youngest lived with their families and Bà Túy in this house. Hồng, her husband Vinh, and their daughter shared one room of their own, and the family of Vinh's brother shared another. Hồng poured hot water from the thermos into the teapot and placed three tiny cups on the table in front of us.

Hằng asked Hồng if she had been granted maternal leave from her job as a kindergarten teacher. Hồng told us that she had, but that she hoped to resume her work soon. She felt restless and bored staying at home; in order to allow her to rest after the abortion, her husband had taken over all daily chores in their family, and there was nothing for her to do. She appreciated his care for her, but she also longed to go back to work and to an ordinary life. A few minutes into our conversation, a tall man arrived, carrying a bag with canned soft drinks and biscuits. In her field notes, Hằng wrote: "Chính is an experienced person and the eldest of the brothers. So he takes care of important family matters. Hồng seemed as if she wanted him to be present." My own observations resembled Hằng's, I wrote: "Hồng clearly expected Chính to come and to take the lead in the talk with us, and he did." Placing the soft drinks on the table, Chính went out to call our driver to come in and join us. Soon after, one of the neighbours, an elderly woman, entered the room, as did several other people, including Hồng's husband Vinh, his younger brother, and Hồng's mother and mother-in-law. Shortly after Chính's arrival, the room was full of people. "We felt a warm and welcoming atmosphere in this family," Hằng wrote in her field notes.

Hằng opened our conversation about the abortion by asking, "How did you organize [the funeral] for the child?" Chính replied by describing his and his family's fears that the deceased fetus might keep haunting its parents, refusing to leave them in peace: "I buried the child and I took care of everything. Hồng and Vinh were not allowed to see the child. Our elders say that if the parents see it, the child will keep following them. The next time they have a child, it will return to them. We feared that this child would keep haunting my brother and his wife, so I had to take care of everything." Later in the conversation, Chính told us in more detail about these fears. In Vietnam, he said, people hold that if a child dies at a very young age, during pregnancy or infancy, it will be reborn, either to the same or to another woman. If the child is born to the same woman, it will suffer from the same weaknesses that it was born with the first time. If a child is born disabled or disfigured, therefore, it is important to prevent it from being reborn to the same woman. To ensure this, people hold, it is of vital importance that the parents do not show their love for their child: if they do, the child will never leave them, but will keep hovering around them, returning in subsequent pregnancies (see Gammeltoft 2010). In the case of Hồng and Vinh, therefore, their elders did not allow them to see the fetus after the abortion or to take part in the funeral.

"How about the first time you lost a pregnancy," Hằng asked Hồng, "what did you do with the fetus after the abortion?" Hồng then told us about the first pregnancy loss she had suffered, at five months' gestation. The abortion had happened unexpectedly, and relatives conducted the funeral in a quick and simple manner. The fetus was buried outside the local commune health clinic. There is a plot of land there, Hồng explained, that is used only to bury children who die before birth: "People don't want to bury them at the ordinary graveyard. They are returning fetuses. They are not children that one can bring up." Hồng's second pregnancy also ended abruptly: she gave birth preterm, at seven months' gestation, in the yard outside the obstetrics hospital in Hanoi. The child died immediately, and unaware of the cultural prohibition against this, Vinh, who had been travelling when the first pregnancy loss occurred, took the child home himself. It was buried at the village burial ground. "Later," he said, "I realised that according to our elders, the parents should not see the child. But at the time I did not know this, so I took the child home." The third pregnancy loss took place at only three months' gestation. Of these four pregnancy losses, Hồng said, the most recent one was the most difficult and the one that had left the deepest impression on her. "This one makes me more worried about the future. If I get pregnant again, will the next child be disabled too?"

Listening to Hồng's story, I wondered whether what made the last pregnancy loss the most emotionally taxing one was not also the fact that there was deliberation involved? Whereas the first three abortions had occurred spontaneously, the fourth loss was willed – Hồng and her family had made an active decision to have this pregnancy terminated. Although the fetus suffered from anencephaly, which meant that even if the pregnancy were carried to term, this child would not be able to live for more than a few hours after the delivery, it seemed that Hồng and her family had the impression that the child might have lived if they had opted to keep the pregnancy. The decision they had made, therefore, concerned whether or not to select this potential child for life. This made me interested in hearing more about the family's ethical deliberations, so I asked, "When you came to your decision after the scan, what were your thoughts about the moral aspects?" In response to this question – which I had posed looking at and expecting an answer from Hồng – her brother-in-law immediately spoke out. "Nobody wanted this to happen," he said, his voice trembling. "But it can be impossible to avoid a difficult fate. This child was already fully formed, a human being, so our family felt very worried. In terms of emotion, we felt so sorry." Leaning back in his chair, Chính indicated that this was all he had to say. The room fell silent. Then Vinh took the floor, explaining that all family members – Hồng and himself, their parents and siblings – had concurred that an abortion was necessary: "We immediately agreed on the abortion," he said. "This was such a painful moment. But allowing the child to live would have been even more painful. The child would have suffered and we would have suffered…". His voice trailed off. Hồng broke the silence, saying, "We all agreed."

Yet behind the family consensus on the necessity of an abortion, I sensed, uncertainties hovered. *Had* this been the right decision? *Could* they have decided otherwise? *Should* they have decided otherwise? I traced this uncertainty in silences and trembling voices; in the very certainty with which Hồng and her relatives insisted on the necessity of the abortion; in the way that they immediately dismissed the thought that they could have kept the pregnancy, closing down any further conversation on this; in Chính's reluctance to elaborate on his observation that this child-to-be had been, as he said, "fully formed, a human being". Conscience questions seemed, I sensed, to threaten to undermine the certainty regarding their decision that Hồng and her relatives strove to convey to us.

When I look back at our conversation with this Hanoian family, I can see in embryonic form the analytical themes that we later developed further. "Reproductive decision-making" became one of our main analytical themes, a theme that Hằng addressed in her master's (Trần 2005) and her PhD thesis (Trần 2011); that several other team members wrote articles about; and that was central to the book I published ten years later (Gammeltoft 2014). In the next section I look closer at the development of key concepts in our research, focusing on the ways in which collaborative relations were placed at the heart of this conceptual work.

Spaces of reflection

On our way home in the car after our visit to Hồng's family, Hằng and I talked. We discussed the fears of being haunted that Hồng's family had expressed, and the ideas that fetuses or children who die at a young age may be reborn, making a more felicitous entry the next time they enter the world. Through this brief discussion in the car, Hằng and I not only summed up a day's work, we also started conceptualizing what was at stake for women in Hồng's situation. A strong sense of attachment to family and local community seemed central, as did the questions of conscience that abortion-seeking women and their relatives often appeared to struggle with. Perhaps their fears of being haunted, I suggested to Hằng, could be seen as instantiations of conscience questions; as if their feelings of having done wrong were embodied in the spectral fetus that they imagined might keep hovering around them?

In ethnographic work, analysis and theory building are on-going endeavors that are integrated into the process of fieldwork rather than taking place when data collection is completed. Through reflections on fieldwork observations, the concepts and theories that sustain the research are constantly developed and refined (e.g., Emerson et al. 2011). In our research in Vietnam, we knew from the beginning that we were interested in processes of decision-making around selective abortions, but the analytical ideas that we pursued did not take full form until we were well into the fieldwork. The specific shape that these ideas took developed out of collective discussions such as those that took place during our visit to Hồng and her family; what happened in these arenas was not only joint data collection, but also joint theorization in the sense discussed by Joanne Rappaport. Pondering how collaborative ethnography can contribute to theoretical innovation, Rappaport (2008: 4–5) points out that collaboration holds the potential to contribute to co-theorization:

By co-theorization, I mean the collective production of conceptual vehicles that draw upon both a body of anthropological theory and upon concepts developed by our interlocutors; I purposefully emphasize this process as one of theory building and not simply coanalysis in order to highlight the fact that such an operation involves the creation of abstract forms of thought similar in nature and intent to the theories created by anthropologists, although they partially originate in other traditions and in non-academic contexts. Understood in this sense, collaboration converts the space of fieldwork from one of data collection to one of co-conceptualization.

In Rappaport's work in Colombia, she and her local colleagues created a conceptual framework revolving around an inside/outside opposition that helped them to comprehend the dynamics of indigenous politics. In Vietnam, my colleagues and I developed a way of thinking about reproductive decision-making that included not only the openly expressed aspects of people's actions and preferences, but also the more subdued and silenced aspects of the decisions that people made when confronted with devastating biomedical information. It was a local concept that led us to this shadow side of human action: the term *ám ảnh*, to haunt or be haunted. This term came up frequently in our conversations with people – it was used to denote pregnant women's fears that if they saw, or heard, something unsettling while they were pregnant, this could leave a lasting imprint on their fetus; it was used to describe people's fears of never being able to forget violent or morally troublesome experiences; and it captured anxieties that the souls of the deceased might continue to haunt the living, refusing to leave them in peace (Gammeltoft 2014). As the case of Hồng's family illustrates, fears that souls of the deceased might continue to "hang around" were particularly vivid in the case of second trimester pregnancy terminations; such fetuses, people imagined, might stay around forever as spectral presences in their parents' lives, angry, sorrowful, and restless.

When making the decision to terminate their pregnancy, all women engaged in open and explicit discussions with family members and health care providers. Like Hồng, they listened to the advice they received from others, and many women seemed to feel that in making their decision, they also made a commitment to the social communities they were part of, acting as a good wife, sister-in-law, community member, or patient (Gammeltoft 2007). Yet beneath this social connection and commitment, more subdued social figures always seemed to hover. Despite the "rightness" of their decision, women felt, a second trimester abortion was also somehow "wrong". The child they had denied a life, they feared, might keep haunting them forever. Social attachment, in other words, had an underside: there was always a remainder, something that didn't fit in, something ghostly that kept intruding and disturbing. This compelled us to see reproductive decision-making as not only a matter of attachment, but also of detachment; of conscious efforts to separate oneself from something or someone. In coming to their decisions, women tied themselves into larger social collectives, of family, kin, and nation, but in order to do this, there were other, and less visible social bonds that they had to deliberately "release" or "kill" (*hóa kiếp*); the bonds that connected them to the child that they did not have. In this way, drawing on local concepts, my Vietnamese colleagues and I rethought the notion of reproductive decision-making, arguing that this concept must be extended to include not only socially acknowledged strivings for attachment and connection, but also a more subdued and shadowy world of loss and separation. Our initial interest in reproductive decision-making, in other words, developed into an analytical framing of decision-making as a question of human efforts to strike a balance between attachment and detachment, connection and disconnection.

The analytical journey that we undertook began during field visits such as the one that Hằng and I paid to Hồng's family. During this visit, Hằng and I pursued a shared, general research agenda, but each of us also had more specific interests that oriented our questions and interactions with Hồng and her relatives. As the above case description illustrates, my questions tended to focus on people's inner lives, on their thoughts and moral deliberations, while Hằng was more interested in the rituals that people turned to in order to cope with the major life disruption posed by a selective abortion. The questions I raised were perhaps influenced by the attention to inner moral life that is so predominant in Christian cultural tradition, while Hằng's questions seemed to be inspired by Buddhism's emphasis on transitions and connections between "this world" and "the other". These differing avenues of approach brought us into other analytical spaces than each of us could have reached on her own; the combination of my focus on inner life and Hằng's focus on ritual interactions helped us to see the double-ness in our interlocutors' lives, to capture the tension between socially acknowledged efforts to tie oneself into specific communities and forces and connections that lie beyond immediate social horizons. Together, in other words, we were "multi-sighted" (Whyte 2014: vii); combining our different points of attention helped us to build a fuller picture of what was at stake in the situation. Throughout the research, moreover, my Vietnamese colleagues and I took up different structural positions: as a foreigner, I was seen by our interlocutors as a "cultural outsider", a person who could legitimately ask basic questions about things that seemed given to everyone else. Being Vietnamese, in contrast, my colleagues were regarded as "cultural insiders" whose questions and reactions indicated that they knew this cultural world well. In methodological terms, this was an advantage, as it allowed us to ask people to elaborate on what to them were cultural givens, at the same time as it enabled us to go along with them on well-trodden cultural paths. Together, in short, my Vietnamese colleagues and I seemed to be seen as culturally double creatures; as octopuses who could engage both from the inside and the outside with the social worlds that people brought us into.

Spaces of emotion

The research we conducted was not only conceptually challenging, but also emotionally and ethically so. We investigated research questions such as: How are morally demanding decisions regarding "defective" fetuses made? How do women and their relatives cope with the loss of a wanted pregnancy at a late stage of gestation? How are fetal remains handled after a late-term abortion? We addressed these sensitive questions in several different sites: in the 3D scanning room where women came for "malformation scans"; in the homes of women whose pregnancies had proceeded without complications; in the antenatal care rooms where women were counselled when a fetal problem was found; and during the family gatherings that arose in people's homes when we visited women whose fetuses had been defined as abnormal. In many cases, women and their families needed time to think before deciding whether to keep or to terminate an affected pregnancy. In those cases, our visit to the family coincided with the existentially fraught moment in which people found themselves balancing between life and death, deeply uncertain about whether to allow or to deny this potential child an existence. These were *ethical moments* in Jarrett Zigon's sense, moments that occur "when some event or person intrudes into the everyday life of a person and forces her to consciously reflect upon the appropriate ethical response" (Zigon 2009: 262). Often, as in Hồng's case, the loss that people confronted made them recall previous losses; losses of children or children-to-be, of love or life opportunities.

The questions that we discussed with people were, in other words, intensely demanding and painful. All the women we met were pregnant with children they had wanted to have, and being informed at a relatively advanced stage of the pregnancy that something was wrong with this fetus threw them into an acute moral and emotional crisis. This crisis seemed to be deepened by two things in particular. First, the fact that they had seen their fetus in the scanning image, "fully formed" with arms, legs, and discernible facial features, seemed to make the women feel more attached to it. This, they felt, was their child; it belonged to them. Second, the fact that the women themselves had to decide whether or not to keep the pregnancy seemed to place an enormous moral burden on them. Even though physicians at the maternity hospital would often offer quite directive advice, the final decision was always placed in the hands of the woman and her relatives. The crisis that this moral plight threw women into was often a prolonged one; when the abortion was over, or when their child had been born, many continued to struggle with conscience questions of various kinds. Had the abortion decision been the right one? Could it be justified? Or, in cases where the pregnancy ended in the birth of a disabled child: Had it been wrong of them to keep the pregnancy, to bring this compromised child into the world?

These fieldwork encounters were, in short, not only spaces of reflection, but also of intense and tumultuous human sentiment. The women we met found themselves at the "edge of existence" (Lester 2013); the existential pain and distress that they experienced often seemed to take them into zones of being that lay beyond that which could be immediately or easily communicated through language. Since they were sensitive and painful, one could have imagined that women would feel most comfortable talking about these questions under more private circumstances, in one-on-one conversations. This, however, was not what we found. On the contrary, we had the impression that it was easier for most women to talk about emotionally upsetting experiences in a situation where they were surrounded by kin, as if the presence of family members helped them to bear the pain of these events and to make it to some extent communicable. Being in the company of the people with whom they lived their daily lives seemed to offer women comfort, helping them to gain a momentary existential foothold at a disruptive and uncertain moment of their lives. In Vietnam, emotion is often described as something to be shared; people attend funerals to "share the sadness" (*chia buồn*) with the bereaved, and they often stress the pleasures of sharing with others the joys and sorrows of their lives (*chia sẻ vui buồn*). The interviews we conducted seemed to be placed within this cultural tradition of emotional sharing; their collective nature turned our interviews into social platforms for emotional exchange.

Being more than one researcher in the field, we found, made it easier for us to create social spaces in which people found it possible to recall and to some extent share intimate and troublesome personal experiences. As Hồng's case illustrates, the interviews we conducted in people's homes often developed from an initial meeting with one woman into lively group discussions in which both family members and neighbours took part. Starting as a private conversation with an individual person, these meetings became communal social arenas that people filled with vivid conversation, debate, and interaction. Although such group sessions might in principle also have developed in research conducted by a solitary anthropologist, the fact that we were always two or three in the field seemed to stimulate these group gatherings, as if our "group-ness" encouraged and condoned our informants' "group-ness". The stories we heard were often co-told by women and their relatives; besides creating an arena for emotional sharing, the active participation of family and community members also seemed to help the women to piece together a coherent narrative out of disjointed and fragmented emotional strands. The process they had been through – the detection of the fetal problem, the decision, the abortion – had often been swift and emotionally chaotic. In the joint family conversations that our research turned into, it seemed, the women pulled together the threads of their life again, and their relatives helped them to do this. The collective nature of the interviews we conducted seemed to facilitate this process, supporting the co-production of stories that helped people to interpret and cope with troublesome events. As Linda C. Garro and Cheryl Mattingly (2000: 1) note: "Creating a narrative, as well as attending to one, is an active and constructive process – one that depends on both personal and cultural resources."

In this emotional space, my Vietnamese co-researchers and I were, again, placed in structurally different positions. Often, the people we met seemed to expect local researchers such as Hằng to be able to follow their emotional intuitions and reactions; being Vietnamese, they seemed to assume, there were certain things that local researchers would understand without much elaboration. One of these things was the anxiety that haunted many women during their pregnancies. As Hồng's story illustrates, pregnancy was, for many women, a state of constant vigilance and anxiety. Due to her history of reproductive losses, Hồng had particular reasons to be worried, but her worries were far from unique. Practically all women we met expressed anxieties about how their pregnancies would end, and yet the depth of these anxieties did not become clear to me until several months into the research. When talking about the value of obstetrical ultrasound, for instance, women would often explain that this technology enables one to *see* the child. It took several months before I realized that this sentence referred to more than the pleasure of meeting one's child-to-be face-to-face – "seeing", as our interlocutors used this term, meant seeing if the fetus had any disabilities. When Chi, as mentioned at the beginning of this chapter, insisted that there were questions we could not ask, it was because she had lived long enough in Vietnam to know of the enormous power held by this anxiety. Being relatively new in Vietnam, I had not yet fathomed the intensity of this anxiety. As Renato Rosaldo (1993) has described so vividly in his classical essay on grief and rage, as ethnographers we sometimes simply do not possess the life experience that is required in order to fully grasp what our interlocutors are telling us. It was only with the sudden death of his own wife, Rosaldo writes, that he understood the connections between grief and rage that Ilongot people had long tried to make him see: "My life experience had not as yet provided the means to imagine the rage that can come with devastating loss" (1993: 4). During our fieldwork in Hanoi, people's experiences resonated in different ways with our own life experiences; it sometimes took time for me to grasp the full force and implications of the emotional experiences that people shared with us and that my Vietnamese colleagues seemed to comprehend more easily and immediately. These different positions enabled us, then, to convey emotional comprehension and non-comprehension at the same time; my status as a foreigner allowed us to invite people to elaborate on their feelings in more detail, at the same time as my colleagues' being Vietnamese allowed us to show an insider's familiarity with the affective dilemmas in which women and their relatives found themselves.

Concluding thoughts

In this chapter, I have offered glimpses into an ethnographic research process, showing how collaborative teamwork shaped conceptual and emotional dimensions of the field research we conducted on selective reproduction in Vietnam. I have shown how the specific and differing life experiences that we brought with us to the research allowed my Vietnamese colleagues and me to pay attention to different things and to respond in different ways to our interlocutors' emotional expressions. The value of this multiplicity of perspectives was crystallized in the research seminars where we shared insights and reflections, doubt and hesitations; these seminars became fertile ground for the development of methodological and analytical ideas.

When using the term "collaboration" in this chapter, I have referred to collaboration among colleagues, and, more specifically, to collaboration among colleagues of different nationalities. What particularly enriched our research, it seemed, was that my colleagues were Vietnamese and I was Danish. In making this observation, I do not want to suggest that there were inherent and fixed cultural differences between us. But the fact that we had grown up and lived most of our lives in different social settings – Hanoi and Copenhagen, respectively – obviously shaped our cognitive and emotional approaches and responses to fieldwork events. In other research teams, other differences among team members – such as age, gender, class, ethnicity, or sexual orientation – may prove salient. As Rosaldo notes, "The ethnographer, as a positioned subject, grasps certain human phenomena better than others. He or she occupies a position or structural location and observes with a particular angle of vision… The notion of position also refers to how life experiences both enable and inhibit particular kinds of insight" (1993:19).

But our being of different national origins, and based in the global South and North respectively, also shaped our research in more unfortunate ways. During the three years of fieldwork, my Vietnamese colleagues and I worked on a relatively equal footing, each of us contributing to the research by posing questions, reflecting on observations, and writing up findings. After the fieldwork was completed, however, the differences between our positions in global academic arenas became more apparent: my – relatively privileged – working conditions at a Danish university allowed me time to write and publish several additional publications, whereas my colleagues in Vietnam were compelled by economic and institutional circumstances to turn to new and income-generating projects. Our possibilities for continued academic work with this ethnographic material were, in other words, shaped by our differing global positions and economic conditions. The joint fieldwork of collegial sharing and cooperation that we strove to conduct was embedded in a larger terrain of global academic inequalities; although these inequalities were rendered relatively invisible during fieldwork, they manifested clearly after it ended. On a more positive note, however, it is important to point out that this and other collaborative projects involving North- and South-based researchers can also be seen as modest contributions towards a more equal world of research; despite the uneven academic playing fields within which my Vietnamese colleagues and I operated, our shared work seemed to strengthen the research capacities of all team members. After this project ended, Chi, Toàn, Hạnh, and Hằng attained PhD scholarships and completed PhD theses on themes close to our research topic, and today Toàn and Hạnh draw routinely on the ethnographic research skills that they acquired during this fieldwork when they, as senior researchers at their home institution, train new generations of students and researchers. The collaboration that we undertook seemed, in short, to become a vital part of continued academic trajectories for us all.

References

Bùi Kim Chi (2005). Quyết Định Đối Với Thai Dị Tất: Vai Trò Của Các Thành Viên Gia Đình (The Role of Family Members in Decision-Making when a Fetus is Anomalous). *Khoa Học Về Phụ Nữ* (*Journal of Women's Studies*) 5(72): 35–42.

Đỗ Thi Thanh Toàn, Nguyễn Thị Thúy Hạnh, Nguyễn Huy Bạo, and Tine Gammeltoft (2005). Tư Vấn Trong Thời Kỳ Mang Thai: Một Việc Làm Thiết Thực cho Những Hoàn Cảnh Thai Bất Thường (Counselling for Pregnant Women: An Important Task when a Fetus is not Normal). *Tạp Chí Nghiên Cứu Y Học* (*Journal of Medical Research*) 39(6): 90–96.

Emerson, Robert M., Rachel I. Fretz, and Linda L. Shaw (2011). *Writing Ethnographic Fieldnotes*. Chicago, IL: University of Chicago Press.

Field, Les and Richard G. Fox, eds. (2007). *Anthropology Put to Work*. Oxford: Berg.

Gammeltoft, Tine M. (2007). Prenatal Diagnosis in Postwar Vietnam: Power, Subjectivity and Citizenship. *American Anthropologist* 109(1): 153–163.

Gammeltoft, Tine M. (2010). Between Remembering and Forgetting: Maintaining Moral Motherhood after Late-Term Abortion. In: Andrea Whittaker, (ed.) *Abortion in Asia: Local Dilemmas, Global Politics*, pp. 56–77. New York: Berghahn Books.

Gammeltoft, Tine M. (2014). *Haunting Images: A Cultural Account of Selective Reproduction in Vietnam*. Berkeley, CA: University of California Press.

Garro, Linda C. and Cheryl Mattingly (2000). Narrative as Construct and Construction. In: Cheryl Mattingly and Linda C. Garro (eds), *Narrative and the Cultural Construction of Illness and Healing*, pp. 1–49. Berkeley, CA: University of California Press.

Gottlieb, Alma (1995). Beyond the Lonely Anthropologist: Collaboration in Research and Writing. *American Anthropologist* 97(1): 21–25.

Gujar, Bhoju Ram and Ann Grodzins Gold (1992). From the Research Assistant's Point of View. *Anthropology and Humanism* 17(3/4): 72–84.

Kemper, Robert V. and Anya Peterson Royce (2002). *Chronicling Cultures. Long-Term Field Research in Anthropology*. Walnut Creek, CA: Altamira Press.

Lassiter, Luke Eric (2005). Collaborative Ethnography and Public Anthropology. *Current Anthropology* 46(1): 83–106.

Lester, Rebecca (2013). Back from the Edge of Existence: A Critical Anthropology of Trauma. *Transcultural Psychiatry* 50(5): 753–762.

Madden, Raymond (2010). *Being Ethnographic. A Guide to the Theory and Practice of Ethnography*. Los Angeles, CA: Sage.

Nguyễn Thị Thuý Hạnh, Nguyễn Huy Bạo, and Tine Gammeltoft (2005). Siêu Âm Chẩn Đoán Thai Sớm Tại Thành Thị Việt Nam: Liệu Dịch Vụ Này Có Bị Lạm Dụng? (Ultrasound Scanning in Urban Vietnam: Is this Service being Misused?) *Tạp Chí Y Học Thực Hành* (*Journal of Practical Medicine*) 530(11): 34–37.

Rappaport, Joanne (2008). Beyond Participant Observation: Collaborative Ethnography as Theoretical Innovation. *Collaborative Anthropologies* 1: 1–31.

Rosaldo, Renato (1993). *Culture and Truth: The Remaking of Social Analysis*. Boston, MA: Beacon Press.

Sanjek, Roger (1993). Anthropology's Hidden Colonialism: Assistants and their Ethnographers. *Anthropology Today* 9(2): 13–18.

Stocking, George W., Jr. (1983). The Ethnographer's Magic: Fieldwork in British Anthropology from Tylor to Malinowski. In: George W. Stocking (ed.) *Observers Observed: Essays on Ethnographic Fieldwork*, pp. 70–120. Madison, WI: University of Wisconsin Press.

Trần Minh Hằng (2005). *Ultrasound Scanning for Fetal Malformations in Hanoi Obstetrical and Gynecological Hospital, Vietnam: Women's Reproductive Decision-Making.* Master's thesis. University of Copenhagen.

Trần Minh Hằng (2011). *Global Debates, Local Dilemmas: Sex-Selective Abortion in Contemporary Vietnam.* PhD thesis. Australian National University.

Whyte, Susan Reynolds, ed. (2014). *Second Chances: Surviving AIDS in Uganda.* Durham, NC: Duke University Press.

Zigon, Jarrett (2009). Within a Range of Possibilities: Morality and Ethics in Social Life. *Ethnos* 74(2): 251–276.

3

WORK PRACTICE ETHNOGRAPHY

Video ethnography in maternity settings

Kajsa Brimdyr

> Making work visible – discovering and describing how people accomplish their tasks, how work actually gets done – reveals what was previously hidden, albeit in plain view. As work practice analysts, our job is to make unbiased observations despite business goals or technology design requirements. If we do our job well, our insights are obvious in retrospect, but by making those insights visible, they become a resource, and we are able to build on them.
>
> Margaret H. Szymanski and Jack Whalen in *Making Work Visible* (2011)

Much of an ethnographer's work helps the invisible to become visible. Work practice ethnographies focus on using the principles of ethnography for the pragmatic and practical design of seeing the work in an unbiased way. This provides an opportunity to value the existing and yet make change for improvements within an institutional setting. Work that is invisible may not be optimally valued – and we measure what we value. Ethnography has often been used as a means to provide "adequate representation of groups who have been somewhat marginalized" (Neyland 2008, p. 5) – bringing their work to light. Therefore, ethnography lends itself to the investigation of birth – often invisible work done primarily by women; recent ethnographies have explored the experiences of the mother, baby and hospital staff (two of my favorite examples: Jordan 1993, Dykes 2006). This chapter will focus on the use of video ethnography to design and implement change within labour and delivery wards in Egypt, Sweden, Romania, and the United States. Video ethnography, combined with education and interaction analysis workshops, offers a rapid method of making sustainable change.

Work practice ethnography

Ethnography has become increasingly popular for qualitative researchers as a method of conducting research. As these adaptations grow and ethnography is used in an ever-growing variety of settings, "we will continue to witness the adjustment of conventional ethnographic methods to the requirements of research..." (Jordan 2009, cited in Gluesing 2009, p. 27). One specific application of ethnography is in the study of workplaces. This type of study grew out of the work of Lucy Suchman and her team at Xerox PARC and IRL in the late 1980s and 90s. The group, Work Practice and Technology, "anchored ethnographic methodology within the organization" (Szymanski & Whalen 2011, p. 3). This is important, Suchman explains, because "the way in which people work is not always apparent. Too often, assumptions are made as to how tasks are performed rather than unearthing the underlying work practices" (Suchman 1995).[1] What people say they do is often different from their actual actions. Work practice ethnographies illuminate the "human agency embedded in the everyday actions and interactions of people doing work in various organizational positions and settings" (Engeström & Middleton 1994). Ethnographic workplace studies focus on the work, people and interactions that happen in a work site. With its basis in ethnomethodology, "the purpose of an ethnographic approach is not so much to show *that* work is socially organized (which is rather easy) but to show *how* it is socially organized" (Bentley et al. 1992).

Ethnography for a work site study emphasizes the generation of a descriptive understanding of the work focusing on the member's point of view. The context of the work practice and the work site, both in terms of the natural setting and the holism of the interactions, are central to ethnographic work site studies. The practice of ethnography consists of two elements: *field observations* – direct observation and informal interviews; and a *product* – often written text highlighting patterns, offering design suggestions or other observations. But what is the role of an ethnographic study?

One view is that "the primary goal of research is, and must remain, the production of knowledge" (Hammersley & Atkinson 1995). A second view is that research, and thereby ethnographic studies, should lead to improved practical problem-solving. In terms of work site ethnographic studies, the role of the ethnographer is often to gain insights into design, product, or barriers (Szymanski & Whalen 2011, pp. 9–10). Whatever the role, the methods of ethnography aim to develop contextual, *in situ* descriptions of the activities, interactions, and patterns of a community. A practical application of the methodology encourages the contextual understanding of work sites, and the *in situ* analysis of work practice, with the aim of improving design.

The purpose and practice of video ethnography

When studying contextually based work practice, video is a natural medium for documentation of real-life situations and locations. It allows for the collection of more data during rich experiences than simple observation or field notes would provide, with the added benefit of being able to review a scenario which "greatly enhance[ed] the range and precision of the observations [that could be] made" (Heritage & Atkinson 1984).

The practice of video ethnography is similar to the practice of conventional ethnography, in that it is comprised of two main elements: a period of field work and a development of product of those observations. With work practice ethnography, and specifically, with video ethnography used in the workplace, video becomes a vital tool for both the field work and the design of practical change.

Field work focuses on "the routine ways in which people make sense of the world in everyday life" (Hammersley & Atkinson 1995). The ethnographer becomes a participant observer – involved with the daily activities of the people who are being studied. Ethnography is grounded in the "fundamental observational and analytical methodologies of participant observation and interviewing" (Rijsberman 2009, p. 77). In anthropologically based ethnography, this usually involves an extended period of time during which the ethnographer becomes immersed in the culture and the lives of the people being studied. In work practice ethnographies, these periods of field work can be less immersive – involving studying people in a specific part of their day: during work, and in a specific location of their daily life: the work site.

Video ethnography involves the use of video in the context of the field work. It does not replace direct observations, informal interviews or other data-gathering aspects of ethnography. Instead, it provides a method to aid observations during fieldwork. Video can be used in many ways – to record interviews, site-specific interactions, or to shadow an individual or artifact's path. In this way, the use of video provides a reliable, reusable tool for the ethnographer to record observations to use later in the interpretation and analysis phase.

The use of video in ethnography has drawbacks as well. The video recording is limited because of the stationary focus of the lens. Occurrences that happen outside of the viewpoint of the camera are lost. Since the video can only record the view of the lens, other sensory features of a site, such as smell, touch, and feel, are lost. The video alone can lose the context of the moment – a central underpinning of ethnography. An ethnographer who uses video must also preserve the external context of the video, in terms of history, politics, and situations, that occur before the video begins, after it ends, and outside of the view of the lens. In this way, the other fieldwork techniques, such as field notes and informal interviews, are significant as a framework for the use of video.

The second element of any ethnography is traditionally the written text of the observations. An ethnographic report is not meant to be simply a recording of data collected, although it often does include "a description of the activities and practices of those studied" (Blomberg et al. 1993, p. 125). Instead, and more importantly, ethnography expects a descriptive reportage that provides an interpretation of the activities observed and described. This interpretation often includes an understanding of the patterns, barriers, values, and efforts of the participants. It may reveal what was "hidden, albeit in plain view... If we do our jobs well, our insights are obvious in retrospect, but by making those insights visible, they become a resource, and we are able to build on them" (Szymanski & Whalen 2011, p. 1).

The understanding of the patterns and processes that come to light through an ethnographic study can be used for more than an academic inquiry. Instead, they can be used for process or design change, or as Brun-Cotton describes them, "ethnographically informed insights for specific institutional interests" (Brun-Cottan 2009, p. 164). For example, a team at Kaiser Permanente used video ethnography in order to understand the experience of the patients in "pivotal points in health care, such as transitions between settings" (Cain et al. 2012). In these cases, the end result may not be a paper, but instead a presentation or a strategy for moving forward. In the case of my work, with PRECESS, the product is the iterative process of sustainable change.

PRECESS

The challenge was to use the strengths of work practice ethnography, and specifically video ethnography, to create long-term, practical change in a medical setting. In this way, the strengths of ethnography would not only be used as a means of understanding the contextual workplace, but also to help iteratively drive its transformation. In this section, I will describe the methodology, PRECESS, which was developed based on the concepts of work practice ethnographies, and utilized video ethnography, to help create sustainable change in the labor and delivery "workplace" of the hospital.

The PRECESS research methodology was developed to drive lasting change through the use of ethnographic methods combined with hands-on expertise. PRECESS stands for Practice, Reflection, Education and training, Combined with Ethnography for Sustainable Success. PRECESS grew out of a three-nation project designed to assist Egypt in re-implementing the WHO/UNICEF Baby Friendly Hospital Initiative (BFHI) in order to revitalize and expand the BFHI. Egypt had been an early implementer of the BFHI but the practice changes of the initiative had not been sustained over time. Healthy Children Project, Inc. was approached to assist in this revitalization.

Healthy Children Project, Inc. is a non-profit research and educational institution dedicated to improving child health outcomes in partnership with governmental, non-governmental, and non-profit agencies. Healthy Children Project conducts research in the United States and abroad, and educates more than 4,000 health care providers a year, as well as partnering with Union

Institute and University for a bachelor's and master's degree in Maternal Child Health: Lactation Consulting. Dr Karin Cadwell, Executive Director of Healthy Children Project, Inc., was an expert on the BFHI, having convened the Baby Friendly Hospital Initiative in the United States.

We hoped to make the BFHI practices a sustainable entity by having an understanding of current practice and best-practice models, evidence-based education, and process-oriented training. This collaboration, between teams from Egypt, the US, and Sweden,[2] provided an opportunity to explore the revised standards and guidelines of the Ten Steps to Successful Breastfeeding of the WHO/UNICEF Baby Friendly Hospital Initiative (BFHI). We decided to focus on Step 4 of the BFHI, which in our experience was the keystone to successful implementation of other steps. Step 4 asks hospitals to provide continuous, uninterrupted skin-to-skin contact between mother and baby beginning immediately after birth and continuing through the first breastfeed.

The implementation of Step 4 of the BFHI may be, literally, a life or death improvement. According to Edmond et al. (2006), continuous skin-to-skin contact with early breastfeeding (Step 4 of the BFHI) could prevent 22 percent of neonatal deaths in developing countries. Continuous skin-to-skin contact in the first hour has been related to improved breastfeeding, fewer supplementations, better temperature regulation of the baby, less crying, improved mother/child bonding, and optimal self-regulation of the infant, and later of the child (Moore, Anderson, & Bergman 2007). Because of these domino effects of getting breastfeeding off to a good start, we decided it was the keystone of the BFHI.

We first gathered an initial baseline of the current labor and delivery practices in Egypt. The team visited, observed, made field notes, took photographs, and recorded video of the current post-birth work practice related to the practices of Step 4 in twelve hospitals and seven primary health centers in seven governorates (two urban, two in Upper Egypt, and three in Lower Egypt) of Egypt. This created a baseline understanding of the practices during the immediate postpartum period throughout Egypt, and gave us a preview of the challenges. None of the hospitals we visited had implemented the internationally agreed best practice of holding a baby skin-to-skin with the mother for the first hour after birth. Our observations were confirmed by the interviews and assessments of the Egyptian Lactation Consultant Association (ELCA), with funding from UNICEF (Abul-Fadl 2008). Within the context of labor, many women arrived at the hospital within two hours of giving birth. The laboring women all stayed in a large room together, until it was decided that birth was imminent. At that point, the woman would be moved to a labor room, where she would climb on a table, give birth, and then be transferred by wheelchair to the recovery room. Mothers who gave birth vaginally would go home within two hours after birth. Mothers who gave birth via cesarean surgery might go to a different part of the hospital, or to an operating theatre connected to the vaginal birth labor ward. Mothers who had cesarean surgery would go home approximately six hours after birth. Many hospitals offered cesareans only under general anesthesia. Some hospitals we visited had a 70 percent cesarean rate.

The hospitals designated to receive the PRECESS intervention were selected by the Egyptian Ministry of Health, and the hospital directors were instructed by the Ministry of Health to accept our assistance in the implementation of best practice. The scope of the project was the labor and delivery ward in the chosen hospital(s), and the purpose was the adaptation of a mother holding a baby skin-to-skin during the first hour after birth. We were given a limited amount of time with each hospital – five consecutive days per hospital, with 24-hour access to the hospital staff during that time.

The translation of theory into sustained practical change can be problematic. Didactic education does not always lead to easy practice change (Christensson et al. 2006). The method of sending one or two staff members away for training (the traditional means of training for the BFHI) does not guarantee policy change or change in hospital practice. Dr. Karin Cadwell (Senior Researcher at HCP) and I strategized about methods of implementation and developed PRECESS, a methodology for driving change that could meet this challenge. We hoped that video ethnography and Interaction Analysis (Jordan & Henderson 1994) combined with expert education and practical application of best practice, would allow us to document the work practice in the hospital and to assist the staff in seeing within their own work the barriers and solutions that, by necessity, would be unique to their situation. We believed PRECESS would allow the vital local context to underlie all solutions, including cultural barriers motivating social, rather than individual, change.

The PRECESS team deliberately included the experts of the intended practice with a work practice ethnographer. Our team consisted of Dr. Ann-Marie Widström, an internationally recognized expert in midwifery and skin-to-skin research from Karolinska Institutet, Sweden, who provided the practical and educational information about the importance of continuous skin-to-skin care in the first hour; Dr. Kristin Svensson, an experienced midwife from Karolinska Hospital, known for her skill at nurturing and mentoring students and families; and myself, with a background in ethnography and maternal child health, focused on understanding work practice as a means of creating meaningful change. This combination of team members allowed a bridge between analytic insights about the ordering of the social world within the hospital setting with the understanding of the work that needed to be accomplished.

This team also allowed us to straddle the gap between insiders and outsiders – an innate tension in ethnographic research. Ethnography balances between participant observation (understandings are the member's point of view of the world they live in) and analytic perspectives (understandings are "constructions that inevitably reflect the socio-historical position and background assumptions of the researchers", Hammersley and Atkinson, 2007, p. 12); between making "the strange familiar... and the familiar strange" (Hammersley and Atkinson, 2007, p. 231). In many respects, two of the team members were insiders –

familiar with hospitals, with labor and delivery wards, with the terminology, clothing, and procedures. It was evident that they were comfortable and familiar with labor and delivery wards; they could integrate in as participant observers within the world we were studying. However, in other respects we were all outsiders: we were not Egyptian, not native speakers, not employees of this hospital, and, of course, not familiar with the work practices of this specific hospital. This balance of insider and outsider lent strength to our ethnographic work. "Without both membership and the capacity to render its taken-for-granted aspects anthropologically strange, it is hard to bring the reasoning and methods that provide for the character of any setting into plain sight" (Tolmie 2011, p. 73).

The PRECESS methodology has five steps. The first step is for the expert in the field to educate the staff about the research behind the new procedure and the concepts associated with implementation. The second step is the practical application of the new procedure, with experts and staff working together, continuing the educational process. The third step is to video tape the evolving process as the hospital staff implement the new procedures. The fourth step is an interaction analysis workshop to review and discuss barriers and solutions. The fifth step is the continuing application of the procedure.

This methodology allowed us to collect data through field work – through informal interview, and video recording of the work in question focusing on the activities of the staff, mother, and baby. Although we were only working in a given setting for five consecutive days, the long-term, multi-location perspective of our use of the methodology (2005–2012, 10 sites) allowed for a sense of immersion in the workplace, giving rise to analytic perspective.

Our goal was to generate a product of the ethnography – a summary of the work practice experience, sifted through by an expert for patterns and design opportunities – that would engender change. Others have documented the importance of "seeing is believing." As Isaacs describes, "we have found that producing these short video summaries of our finding greatly increases the impact of our work, since the videos show rather than tell what we learned, and people find them more engaging than slide sets of documents" (Isaacs 2013, p. 96). However, the product in our case – video segments for use during interaction analysis labs – was specifically for the transitory experience. The segments were designed to be viewed only by the staff members at this hospital, and were seen as a temporary snapshot. The work practice of the next birth would be different, since the staff members had seen, reflected on, and would be adjusting their actions. The constant evolution of the video segments allowed the staff to "see" their progress in a tangible way. These were not a glossy finished product that would be seen by others. Instead, they were a tool that belonged to the staff, and they were eager to make, and see, their progress.

Step one: Educate the staff

Using large group lecture, small group discussion, and informal hallway conversations, we offer numerous opportunities for education to the staff.

On the first day, after meeting with the hospital director, we gather the hospital staff to present an overview of the research about the importance of continuous skin-to-skin contact in the first hour. Research about the advantages of this first hour is presented (Bystrova et al. 2003; 2009; Moore, Anderson, & Bergman 2007) along with education about the baby's nine stages during this time in pictures and video (*Breastfeeding: Baby's Choice* 2007; *Skin to Skin in the First Hour After Birth* 2010; *The Magical Hour* 2011). This forms the foundation for the motivation for implementing best practice, and mirrors the education typically presented about best practices.

We also show video of the practice in action and the specific observable behavior of the baby. Research shows us that babies go through nine distinctive stages during the first hour or so after birth when they are placed skin-to-skin with their mother: the Birth Cry, Relaxation, Awakening, Activity, Rest, Crawling, Familiarization, Suckling, and Sleeping (Widström et al. 2011). By focusing on the instinctive behavior of the baby, rather than the clock, we can illuminate the motivation behind the directive. Step 4 requires the baby to be left with the mother "about an hour until the first breastfeed". This can result in watching the clock, and perhaps helping/forcing the baby to breastfeed. Changing the focus from the time to the baby allows us to see the important work the baby is accomplishing during this short time, and competent behavior of the baby helps to underscore the purpose of the change. Initially we showed Ann-Marie's *Breastfeeding: Baby's Choice* DVD, and then we used the DVD the three of us developed together for this purpose – *Skin to Skin in the First Hour After Birth: Practical Advice for Staff*. Obstetricians, pediatricians, surgeons, anesthesiologists, and nurses are invited to attend.

As we move out of the formal classroom setting and to the labor and delivery/ surgery ward, there are opportunities for one-on-one questions, and we create an environment in the ward where any "down time" is an opportunity for small group discussions. The PRECESS team is always available, always accessible. Since there are different shifts in hospital wards, we strive to be available for all shifts, providing appropriate education about the new process.

Step two: Practical application

Immediately begin to implement the best practice, with guidance from the external experts.

The PRECESS team then demonstrates, with assistance from the staff, the practical application of the procedure. This encourages more questions, as implementation illuminates practical difficulties and questions. The education of the staff continues in the delivery and/or surgery ward. The PRECESS team coaches in the hands-on application of immediate and continuous skin-to-skin contact post vaginal and caesarean births. These external experts provide clinical and practical assistance to achieve the appropriate practice in the current setting, and to mentor the staff during the transition. This step helps to overcome the common cry of resistance – "but it can't be done in *this* setting."

Step three: Record evolving process

Unobtrusively record the implementation of the practice. This provides an opportunity to document the ability to perform the best practice in the context of the environment, and also provides the initial material for the discussion of challenges.

One member of the team, the video ethnographer, unobtrusively records the evolving process by videotaping the activities in the delivery/surgical ward. The video ethnographer has firm knowledge of the practice of skin-to-skin in the first hour after birth as well as background in work practice. The ethnographer records the interactions between staff, the mother, and the experience of the baby.

The small, lightweight, high definition, good-in-low-light video camera we use to document the work practice has an added swivel feature, so we can turn the screen around to view it from a different angle. This had the serendipitous advantage of providing a view of the activity to an extended group. During a cesarean surgery, the screen could be rotated, allowing the surgeons a clear view of a healthy, happy baby moving through the stages of awakening while skin-to-skin on the mother's chest as they continued the operation.

Step four: Interaction analysis workshop

The interaction analysis workshops provide an opportunity to examine the actual actions and reactions, and to discuss the process in a relaxed and thoughtful setting.

Every day the PRECESS team chooses rich segments of video and prepares them for the workshop. These segments could highlight a particular achievement, a barrier, or an idea to generate conversation. The segments represent emerging patterns and roadblocks to be conquered.

Discussion and choosing of a rich segment represents a collaboration between the conceptual idea of outsiders and insiders on the team. It begins with conversations about the experiences thus far, and specific moments and themes that stand out from our field observations. What is the understanding of the practice of the participants who are recorded on the video? At the same time, we are looking of the analytic opportunities – what do we see, as outsiders, that are not obvious to the participants? We then review the segment, to see what the video has captured in comparison to our memories of events. Sometimes we find a rich segment that matches our memories of the event. Other times, we see something on the video that illuminates an aspect of the work practice that we did not notice during our time of observation. These discussions and editing events often occur in the hospital break room, between times of informal education and births, since we were usually available to the hospital 24 hours a day for the five days of the intervention.

The Interaction Analysis workshop is attended by doctors (OB specialists, pediatricians, anesthesiologists, pharmacologists, neonatalogists), nurses (head nurses, staff nurses, student nurses), and administration. There could be other relevant personnel as well, or they could have their own workshop. During an interaction analysis workshop, the video segments are played, and can be stopped at any time with a question or comment from the group. It is possible to rewind the video to review it again. The PRECESS team are available to facilitate discussion, to offer expert opinion, to praise good practice, and to warn about possible dangers. However, all comments are tailored to be constructive, and to be carefully integrated into conversation, not presented in lecture format.

The responsibility for the pace and discussion of the workshop lies with the participants, as they examine their evolving practice and work as a group to solve barriers. This process elicits lively discussion as hospital staff notice barriers on the video, discuss barriers they had been thinking about, but perhaps not sharing, and can see the effectiveness of the process they have begun.

Repeated viewings allow the participants to focus on multiple aspects of the segment – who is standing where and why? What is the apparent experience of the mother? The baby? The OB? The nurse? Others in the room? What are the roles of various tools and artifacts? Workshop participants who are also on the video have the opportunity to share their own memories of the experience, and to enrich the contextual understanding of the short clip. This microanalysis through iterative analysis guides participants through a collaborative process that illustrates the work practice.

Step five: Ongoing application

The ongoing application of the practice, supported by the team, but designed to increase confidence and independence of the hospital staff, exploring the barriers and solutions to the practice over five continuous days.

The staff continue to ask questions and gain education. As more babies are born, the hospital staff continue to apply the procedure. The videotaping continues, with the ability to have more interaction analysis workshops. Most importantly, the staff have learned to discuss and review barriers and solutions to the application of the procedure. This occurs with the experts, and the problem-solving should continue after the experts leave. As invited experts with a limited time to implement change, we felt like we needed to instill in the hospital staff a sense of personal responsibility – not only for the changes to practice, but for the solutions to the barriers that would be discovered only after we had left. Solving the barriers of today simply reveals the barriers of tomorrow. The hospital staff then have the responsibility to continue the process, and to solve the barriers to the process that will arise in the future. It is important not to create a stagnant solution, but to instill a responsibility to promote continuous improvement. This is problem-solving approach is modeled and practiced throughout the five days.

A key component of this method is the basic assumption that the staff members at the site are the experts of their environment – not the outsiders who are brought in. Although these external experts have vital information about research, experience, and practice, the hospital staff are the experts on their hospital – its practice, history, and people. The change needs to grow from within the already-existing environment in order to succeed. External experts can offer information, but in order for that information to be integrated into the hospital's practice for long-term success, the material needs to be embraced by the staff.

Examples: Two cases of PRECESS implementation

We have conducted the PRECESS methodology in many different locations throughout the world. We have worked in a small hospital with 300 births a month and a city hospital with 800 births a day. We have worked at cutting-edge hospitals with every technology possible, and ones with intermittent running electricity. We have conducted this methodology in both resource-rich and resource-poor countries. In every case, the structure of the methodology reveals the similarities of flow of work as well as the unique challenges. In each hospital there is the reward of implementing best practice. In this section, two examples of implementation are elaborated further.

Case 1: Upper Egypt example

This hospital is a rural district hospital in an area of Upper (Southern) Egypt with limited resources. There are approximately 60,000 villagers in the area. The hospital has around 300 births per month. Of these, approximately 50 per month are cesarean births.

Step one: Educate the staff

On the first day, after meeting with the director of the hospital, we gathered the staff including surgeons, obstetricians, pediatricians, nurses, and nursing students. Simultaneous translation was provided. We presented an overview of the research about the importance of continuous skin-to-skin contact in the first hour, and explained that this was a process central to the Egyptian Ministry of Health's goal of revitalizing the BFHI in Egypt. Although we invited questions, there were very few.

Step two: Practical application

After the seminar, we moved immediately to the upper levels of the hospital. There were no vaginal births expected in the next few hours, but a cesarean birth was beginning shortly. The mother was counseled about the importance of skin-to-skin by one of the surgeons who had attended the lecture, consent was obtained from both the mother and her husband, and the cesarean began.

The mother was medicated with spinal anesthesia. The baby was extracted, and immediately placed skin-to-skin on the mother's chest. The staff, many of whom accompanied us to the operating theatre from the education session, were able to watch as the baby gave a birth cry, relaxed, opened his eyes, and went through the documented stages of the first hour while skin-to-skin with the mother. This opportunity to see the actions of the baby – their own baby – was profound. Seeing the video of another baby – in a foreign-looking hospital – does not instill a belief that those actions are reproducible by a baby in Southern Egypt. Seeing their own baby progress through the stages in front of them (clearly not being manipulated by clever video editing) instilled a feeling of awe – "*our* babies can do this."

There was much excitement in the room about the baby – who would usually have been transferred to the nursery immediately after the birth. The external experts mentored the nurses in their new role – watching the baby, keeping it from falling, talking to the mother, keeping the baby's airways clear, etc.

During the operation, the issue of resuscitation arose almost immediately, although it had not been raised in the lecture. At this hospital, all babies had received tracheal suctioning after birth. Mentoring the best practice procedure could be illustrated clearly for a large audience, with a healthy example immediately in front of them who had not received suctioning. This allowed demonstration, later followed by staff education, about the recommended best practices of international agencies, which now do not condone routine suctioning, even for babies with meconium-stained amniotic fluid (Kattwinkel et al. 2010; ACOG 2007).

Step three: Record evolving process

The process of the cesarean and the immediate skin-to-skin contact was recorded onto a hand-held video camera. The video recording was unobtrusive, and did not interfere with the actions and interactions in the room. The intended reason for using the video was for the improvement of the hospital's own practice. It was important to develop trust and rapport with the mothers, fathers, and hospital staff. Permission for videotaping was given by the mother and father, the Ministry of Health, the director of the hospital, and the hospital staff.

Step four: Interaction analysis workshop

On the morning of the third day, after we had worked together on many cesarean and vaginal births for a day and a half, we presented the first interaction analysis workshop. We had chosen three rich segments to discuss. These segments were typical of the evolving process.

During the workshop, which was translated, the interprofessional group of obstetricians, OBs, pediatricians, and nurses immediately began discussing what they saw on the video, which was projected so everyone could see it clearly. Although we moderated the discussion, we allowed the staff to drive and direct it, with conversations jumping from the clothes worn by the mother during labor to the need for pillows so she could see her baby, from the lack of money for supplies to a re-imagining of how one of the nearby rooms could be used for mothers during the first hour.

The workshop provided an opportunity for the staff to gather and see the important changes they had made so far – to see the look on the mother's face as she watched her baby while on the delivery table, to watch the baby wake up and go through the stages during the first hour. The workshop provided "proof" of the small, measurable outcomes that had been accomplished in the short period of time, and motivated the discussion of the next steps. The participants received immediate, satisfying reinforcement of the intervention, as well as affirming the pathway for continued progress.

Step five: Ongoing application

After the workshop, we returned to the delivery room and operating theatre to implement the ideas discussed during the workshop, and to think about the process in practice. The staff problem-solved to find pillows for the mothers, and to allow them enough time post-partum to complete the hour of skin-to-skin time. The nursing students had charts in Arabic with the nine stages that the baby goes through during the first hour, and could help the mother know that the baby wasn't yet ready to nurse, but could direct her see the baby awakening and moving through the stages.

As the project continued throughout the days, the grandmothers in the hospitals (who usually brought the pregnant mother, sat in the laboring room with her, and stayed with her in the recovery room before going home) began to interact with each other about the skin-to-skin babies in the recovery room. As the change swept through the hospital, the recovery room became filled with quiet, skin-to-skin babies, rather than crying babies. Since the laboring room and recovery room were adjacent, many of the "laboring" grandmothers began to visit the "recovery" grandmothers to discover the change. The "recovery" grandmothers, who had been quickly educated by the hospital staff when the mother was returned with the baby to leave them together and watch for the baby's instinctive behavior, would proudly display their clever and accomplished babies for the "laboring" grandmothers. In this way, news about skin-to-skin moved into the wider community – via the recovery room, the laboring room, and then the village. When we visited the Case 1 hospital years later, we heard that the grandmothers were still educating pregnant women about the importance of skin-to-skin immediately after birth. If we had conducted a study, we may have determined that one way to create change would be to involve and educate the local grandmothers! However, this methodology allowed the organic growth of a solution best suited for this specific context.

Measuring sustainability

We were fortunate in Egypt to have a second intervention going on at the same time, and to have a UNICEF funded on-site survey happening within weeks, and then again months, after the interventions. The evaluation of the methodology was completely separate from the intervention. This allowed us to use realistic evaluation to measure the success of the PRECESS intervention (Brimdyr et al. 2012).

While we were conducting the PRECESS methodology at the Case 1 hospital, representatives from five regional hospitals attended a comprehensive 20-hour training at a Ministry of Health facility. This training was conducted by internationally respected faculty, and included the importance of continuous, uninterrupted skin-to-skin in the first hour after birth (Step 4 of the Baby Friendly Hospital Initiative). This type of training – sending a couple of staff members to a respected training program – is a standard method of educating staff.

Four months after the PRECESS intervention at the Case 1 hospital, a national survey revealed that the hospitals that had received the conventional trainings at the teaching hospital could correctly answer questions about the benefits of skin-to-skin and the benefits of early initiation of breastfeeding at better rates than Case 1 hospital. However, when the question concerned implementation – specifically asking "Do your colleagues practice skin-to-skin in the first hour with their patients?" – the results were markedly different. This revealed that even though the staff could answer questions about the importance of continuous, uninterrupted skin-to-skin in the first hour, they were not implementing it in their hospitals. However, 80 percent of staff at the hospital with the PRECESS intervention reported that their colleagues were practicing continuous, uninterrupted skin-to-skin in the first hour, compared with none at all at the other hospitals. The PRECESS methodology allowed hospitals to explore the practical application of the new process, solve the initial challenges to the implementation with on-site assistance, and to learn to identify and solve the barriers to the process, allowing sustainability to the process.

The PRECESS methodology was repeated in five different governorates across Egypt between 2005 and 2011. The selection of PRECESS intervention hospitals focused on teaching hospitals, including one with over 800 births per day. Egypt had a 63 percent decline in newborn mortality from 1990 to 2011, from 20 newborn deaths per 1,000 live births per day to 7 (Save the Children 2013), the third largest decline in the world.

Case 2: Southwestern USA example

This hospital is a non-profit private medical center in a major city in Texas, United States that averages 6,000 births per year, with a 40 percent cesarean rate. In this case, the PRECESS methodology was implemented at the hospital as part of a Quality Improvement project.

Step one: Educate the staff

On the first day, after meeting with the director of the hospital, we gathered the staff including a few obstetricians and pediatricians, but primarily nurses. We presented an overview of the research about the importance of continuous skin-to-skin contact in the first hour, and explained that this was an example of best practice that was currently being implemented as a Quality Improvement project at the hospital. Research about the advantages of skin-to-skin during the first hour was presented along with education about the baby's nine stages during this time, using pictures and video. Although we invited questions, there were very few. This seminar was presented for the day shift, and again for the night shift.

Step two: Practical application

After the seminar, we moved immediately to the labor and delivery ward of the hospital. We systematically conducted informed consent interviews with the mothers on the floor.

The staff at this hospital had previously been informed about the importance of skin-to-skin in the first hour, and self-reported that it was provided to all vaginal birth mothers.

Skin-to-skin was not available to mothers of cesarean surgery because the hospital was having an unrelated issue of maternal hypothermia after surgery. There was extreme concern for introducing a vulnerable baby into an already cold environment and babies born via cesarean surgery were placed into warming cots.

Step three: Record evolving process

We began filming with the first vaginal birth, focusing on the behavior of the baby during the first hour, and were surprised to see that, although the baby went through the initial stages, the baby fell asleep after the birth cry, relaxation, awakening, and activity. Years of experience informed our team that this was not a normal behavior. The second vaginal birth baby filmed at this hospital had a similar pattern – birth cry, relaxation, awakening, activity, sleep. These babies were failing to accomplish the crawling, familiarization and suckling behaviors instinctive during the first hour. We were unable to record and demonstrate the innate behavior of the baby. This new and concerning pattern caused significant discussions with the team. We had never seen this arrested behavior, even after general anesthesia, or other traumatic birth experiences; certainly, never after a calm vaginal birth.

A review of the literature reminded us that babies exposed to a high level of certain medications during labor have limited success with breastfeeding, when measured six weeks later (Beilin et al., 2005). Could this be related?

We edited the video, and conducted an educational in-service with the labor and delivery anesthesia staff on site. We showed video of babies moving through the nine stages while skin-to-skin with mother, as filmed in other hospitals. We then showed the edited video of the arrested behavior of the two babies we had seen on the floor. We presented copies of the research papers implicating specific labor medications with breastfeeding difficulties. We did not push for changes or answers, simply presented information. The anesthesia staff were very interested in the information, and took an active interest in the behavior during the first hour of the babies during the rest of the five days we were there. Although we were not offered any explanation, none of the babies born after we presented the research information had the unusual arrested behavior. This practical, non-judgmental problem-solving is a classic element of PRECESS.

Step four: Interaction analysis workshops

In this hospital, we were given an unused triage room adjacent to the nurses' station to use as our home base. We set up the room with a table and two chairs, and a laptop computer that constantly displayed new clips of the process. Nurses and OBs would stop by the room several times a day, alone or in groups of two, three, or up to ten. They would watch the loop of the rich segment, stopping it to discuss observations. We also conducted more formal workshops, as when the head of Quality Improvement for the hospital visited the floor, and reviewed and discussed a segment with the clinical specialist and several nurse supervisors.

In all of the formal and informal interaction analysis workshops, there was amazement among staff that the babies were accomplishing the nine stages of behavior in their hospital. The context created an increased belief in the theory. As one L&D nurse said when she watched one of their own babies go through the nine stages: "I have been working in Labor and Delivery for 30 years, and I have never seen anything like that!" One nurse confessed that she imagined we had filmed thousands of babies to create the clip we had shown them in the in-service about the innate behavior of the babies.

Step five: Ongoing application

Throughout the five days, we continued to assist with, and video tape, the evolving process. We assisted in the understanding that both mothers and babies are warmer when skin-to-skin with each other, which helped to solve the issue with cesarean hypothermia (Crenshaw et al. 2012). There were both large and small changes, as different types of barriers were approached, discussed, and sometimes solved. Not everything can be solved within five days. The challenge is to create an environment that is dedicated to the practice change, and equipped to work through barriers as they arise.

Measuring sustainability

We were fortunate that the PRECESS Quality Improvement project within the Case 2 hospital was conducted within the framework of a dissertation for a Doctorate of Nursing Practice, using data that the hospital routinely collected before and after the intervention. The student found that the intervention created significant improvement to the implementation of skin-to-skin immediately after birth in the labor and delivery ward. Within the health care system, and within workplace ethnographies, the product will most likely be measured in order to be valued.

Practical challenges to PRECESS

There are practical challenges to engaging in a methodology like PRECESS. Recording the process with video is a critical element of the process, and yet it can be a challenge to gain permission to videotape. In the US, our IRB (Institutional Review Board) requires many extra pages on a consent before researchers are allowed to video mothers and babies. In a litigious society, it can be a challenge to gain permission and the trust of the staff to videotape. Our personal reputations and institutional reputations help to open doors, but this must be augmented with onerous paperwork and permissions before even entering a hospital. The ethnographer earns trust during the process via judicious choice of rich segments which are representative, non-judgmental and ethically secure.

Another practical challenge is that babies arrive 24 hours a day, 7 days a week! The PRECESS team must be available for all shifts in order to capture and mentor practice. This requires an energetic and dedicated team of researchers who are willing and able to commit to this rigorous and intense process.

The personalities of the team are also important. The experts must exhibit a demeanor of humility and care; they must coach, mentor and educate, shifting easily between these roles. Formal education, collegial mentoring, and coaching quietly from a distance, allow the hospital team to maintain control of their space, their process and the safety of their mothers and babies. The team must be both non-judgmental and highly ethical with a clear focus on the directive: the BFHI interpretation of skin-to-skin for healthy mothers and babies.

Creating presence

John Kennell's pioneering work on presence showed that the simple addition of a nursing student in a laboring woman's room decreased the rates of cesarean section (Kennell et al. 1991). There is a significant body of research suggesting that the success of midwives in decreasing cesarean section is related to their very presence – they are an active, involved member of the laboring woman's experience. In many ways, the PRECESS methodology encourages this same type of presence. The ethnographic methodology, introduced by experts, then transferred through the interaction analysis labs and ongoing iterations by and to the members of the community, encourages the members to be *present* in the experience. Being present illuminates the actual work in the environment – the work of the other staff, of the artifacts, of the mother, and of the baby. This presence motivates change as the barriers become visible.

For example, although the PRECESS team highlights the importance of "continuous, uninterrupted" skin-to-skin contact, as highlighted by the BFHI directives, we do not illustrate in the initial lecture the consequences of interruption. And yet, once the process has begun in each location, someone has brought forward the observation of the effect of removing a baby from the mother's chest during the first hour; the baby needs to begin the stages again. For example, if a baby has progressed from the Birth Cry, to Relaxation, Awakening, Activity, and Crawling, and then needs to be removed so that the mother can climb down from the birthing table, when the baby is reunited skin-to-skin with his mother, he invariably will begin at the beginning again at Stage 1. He will Cry, Relax, make small Awakening movements, and so on. However, since babies are only awake for the first hour and a half or so after birth, they have a limited time to progress through these stages and achieve suckling during that time before falling asleep. If a baby is removed from mother, there is a chance he will not be able to progress through the stages before the mandatory Sleep stage. If we, the PRECESS experts, point this out to the hospital staff on the first day, it would seem admonitory: "you must keep them together – or else." By letting the staff discover for themselves, an internal motivation is created for the change in practice. Allowing the important work of the baby to appear in the awareness of the community encourages the active presence of the staff within the activities of the ethnographic work practice site.

This desire to keep the mother and baby together, once the motivation has been created, opens a whole new layer of challenges, ones that the hospital community would not have been prepared to deal with in the first days of the intervention. If the baby must be kept skin-to-skin with the mother, and now the personal observations are driving the desire to see the best possible outcome for the baby, then how do we overcome the need for the mother to move off of the surgery table? This challenge occurs at each site, with the need for a location-specific solution. This challenge is a perfect example of the need for a solution rising out of the knowledge and expertise of the community.

Ethnography develops different relationships than consulting: the knowledge, the expertise of the location being studied, lives with the members. The methodology respects that the solution will grow from the internal, location-specific challenges. We trust that once the members of the community of practice are present in the experience – are seeing the work practice around them – their skills and knowledge of their own setting will illuminate an appropriate, location-specific solution. When the five days of the intervention ends, the sustainability remains because the process belongs to the staff, not to outside consultants. Ethnography innately creates presence – its very process, the questioning and sharing, serves to illuminate work in a new way.

Conclusion

Work practice ethnography is a powerful methodology that expects meaningful workplace transformation and allows multiple contextual pathways for success toward the ultimate goal of sustainable positive change improving the experience and healthy outcome of mothers and babies. A small team of external experts were able to create significant and lasting change in hospital settings using the five-day method of PRECESS – Practice, Reflection, Education and Training, Combined with Ethnography for Sustainable Success. This five-step methodology combines education with practical application, and offers a means to see and change existing barriers, with solutions grounded in local context from the hospital staff. Conducting the same process, with the same team, in different situations, allows the ethnographer to see the value of the replication; the unfolding similarities and differences are allowed and encouraged to be discovered. This methodology does not create generalizable answers. Instead, the context-specific, ethnographic approach embraces the flow of expert-enhanced opportunities for evidence-based practice change.

Notes

1 During the time that this exciting reconceptualizing was occurring in California, I was working at a university in southern Sweden, Hogskolan Karlskrona/Ronneby (later Blekinge Tekniska Hogskolan) with a team led by the visionary Bosse Helgeson with Berthel Sutter, Sara Ericsén, and Björn Andersson, to develop a bachelor's and masters' degree in People, Computers, and Work – a blending of cognitive psychology, software engineering, and work practice. This melding built on the philosophies of grounded theory, ethnomethodology, hermeneutics, participatory design, computer-supported cooperative work, Piaget's epistemology, and software engineering. With so much overlap, it was exciting for the faculty and researchers in the department to work in partnership with the team at Xerox PARC, with Lucy Suchman, Randy Trigg, Jeannette Blomberg, Julian Orr, Brigitte Jordan, and others, to help our students and our faculty to understand and expand this exciting fusion of ethnography and design.
2 This project was a collaboration of Healthy Children Project (USA); Karolinska Hospital, Karolinska Institute's Division of Reproductive, Blekinge Institute of Technology and Perinatal Health Care (Sweden); The Egyptian Lactation Consultant Association, Cairo University's Center of Social and Preventive Medicine, Maternal and Child Health Department in Ministry of Health and Population, Quality Assurance Department in MOHP, and UNICEF (Egypt).

References

Abul-Fadl, A. (2008). Baseline assessment of baby-friendly hospitals in Upper Egypt governorates, prepared by the Egyptian Lactation Consultant Association (ELCA) in consultation with MCH/MOHP-AUH & UNICEF/ECO. Egyptian Lactation Consultant Association.

American Congress of Obstetricians and Gynecologists (ACOG). (2007, Sept). Committee Opinion No. 379: Management of delivery of a newborn with meconium-stained amniotic fluid. *Obstetrics & Gynecology,* 110(3), 739.

Beilin, Y., Bodian, C.A., Weiser, J., Hossain, S., Arnold, I., Feierman, D.E.... & Holzman, I. (2005). Effect of labor epidural analgesia with and without fentanyl on infant breast-feeding: a prospective, randomized, double-blind study. *Anesthesiology,* 103(6), 1211–1217.

Bentley, R., Hughes, J.A., Randall. D., Rodden, T., Sawyer, P., Shapiro, D., & Somerville, I. (1992). Ethnographically-informed systems design for air traffic control. *Conference on Computer-Supported Cooperative Work 1992 Proceedings*. New York: ACM Press.

Blomberg, J., Giacomi, J., Mosher, A., & Swenton-Hall, P. (1993). Ethnographic field methods and their relation to design, in Schuler, D. & Namioka, A., (eds), *Participatory Design: Principles & Practices*. Hillsdale, NJ: Lawrence Erlbaum.

Brimdyr, K. (Producer) (2010). *Skin to skin in the first hour after birth: Practical advice for staff after vaginal and cesarean birth* [DVD]. East Sandwich, MA: Health Education Associates.

Brimdyr, K. (Producer) (2011). *The magical hour: Holding your baby skin to skin for the first hour after birth* [DVD]. East Sandwich, MA: Health Education Associates.

Brimdyr, K., Widström, A.M., Cadwell, K., Svensson, K., & Turner-Maffei, C. (2012). Realistic evaluation of two training programs on implementing skin to skin as a standard of care. *Journal of Perinatal Education,* 21 (3), 149–157.

Brun-Cottan, F. (2009). Doing corporate ethnography as an outsider, in Jordan, B. (ed.), *Advancing Ethnography in Corporate Environments: Challenges and Emerging Opportunities*. Walnut Grove, CA: Left Coast Press.

Bystrova, K., Widström, A.M., Matthiesen, A.S., Ransjö-Arvidson, A.B., Welles-Nyström, B., Wassberg ...& Uvnäs-Moberg, K. (2003). Skin-to-skin contact may reduce negative consequences of 'the stress of being born': A study on temperature in newborn infants, subjected to different ward routines in St. Petersburg. *Acta Paediatrica,* 92(3), 320–326.

Bystrova, K., Ivanova, V., Edhborg, M., Matthiesen, A.S., Ransjö-Arvidson, A.B., Mukhamedrakhimov, R.... & Widström, A.M. (2009). Early contact versus separation: Effects on mother–infant interaction one year later. *Birth,* 35(2), 97–109.

Cain, C., Neuwirth, E., Bellows, J., Zuber, C., & Green, J. (2012). Patient experiences of transitioning from hospital to home: An ethnographic quality improvement project. *Journal of Hospital Medicine.* Retrieved from: http://www.ncbi.nlm.nih.gov/ pubmed/22378714.

Christensson, K., Pettersson, K.O., Bugalho, A., Cunha, M., Dgedge, C., Johansson, E., & Bergström, S. (2006). The challenge of improving perinatal care in settings with limited resources. Observations of midwifery practices in Mozambique. *African Journal of Reproductive Health,* 1, 47–61.

Crenshaw, J.T., Cadwell, K., Brimdyr, K., Widström, A.M., Svensson, K., Champion, J.D... . & Winslow, E.H. (2012). Use of a video-ethnographic intervention (PRECESS Immersion Method) to improve skin-to-skin care and breastfeeding rates. *Breastfeeding Medicine,* 7(2), 69–78. Retrieved from http://www.ncbi.nlm.nih. gov/pubmed/22313390.

Dykes F (2006) *Breastfeeding in Hospital: Midwives, Mothers and the Production Line.* London: Routledge.

Edmond, K.M., Zandoh, C., Quigley, M.A., Amenga-Etego, S., Owusu-Agyei, S., & Kirkwood, B.R. (2006). Delayed breastfeeding initiation increases risk of neonatal mortality. *Pediatrics,* 117(3): e380–6. Retrieved from: http://pediatrics.aappublications. org/content/117/3/e380.

Engeström, Y., & Middleton, D. (eds.). (1994). *Cognition and Communication at Work.* Cambridge: Cambridge University Press.

Gluesing, J. (2009). The power of conventional ethnographic methods, in Jordan, B. (ed.), *Advancing Ethnography in Corporate Environments: Challenges and Emerging Opportunities.* Walnut Grove, CA: Left Coast Press.

Hammersley, M., & Atkinson, P. (1995). *Ethnography: Principles in Practice* (2nd edn). New York: Routledge.

Hammersley, M., & Atkinson, P. (2007). *Ethnography: Principles in Practice* (3rd edn). New York: Routledge.

Heritage, J., & Atkinson, J.M. (Eds.). (1984). *Structures of Social Action: Studies in Conversation Analysis.* Cambridge: Cambridge University Press.

Isaacs, E. (2013). The value of rapid ethnography. In Jordan, B. (ed.), *Advancing Ethnography in Corporate Environments: Challenges and Emerging Opportunities.* Walnut Creek, CA: Left Coast Press.

Jordan, B. (1993). *Birth in Four Cultures.* Long Grove, IL: Waveland Press.

Jordan, B. (2009). Blurring boundaries: The 'real' and the 'virtual' in hybrid spaces. Introduction to special section on knowledge flow in online and offline spaces. *Human Organization,* 68(2), 181–193.

Jordan, B. & Henderson, A. (1994). Interaction analysis: Foundations and practice. *Journal of the Learning Sciences,* 4 (1), 39–103.

Kattwinkel, J., Perlman, J.M., Aziz, K., Colby, C., Fairchild, K., Gallagher, J., ... & Zaichkin, J. (2010, November). Special report: Neonatal resuscitation: 2010 American Heart Association guidelines for cardiopulmonary resuscitation and emergency cardiovascular care. *Pediatrics,* 126 (5), 1400–1413.

Kennell, J., Klaus, M., McGrath, S., Robertson, S., & Hinkley, C. (1991). Continuous emotional support during labor in a US hospital: A randomized controlled trial. *Journal of the American Medical Association.* 265(17), 2197–2201.

Moore, E.R., Anderson, G.C., & Bergman, N. (2007). Early skin-to-skin contact for mothers and their healthy newborn infants. *Cochrane Database of Systematic Reviews.* 18(3). doi: 10.1002/14651858.

Neyland, D. (2008). *Organizational Ethnography.* Thousand Oaks, CA: Sage Publications.

Rijsberman, M. (2009). Ethnography and product design: fixing the future, in Jordan, B. (ed.), *Advancing Ethnography in Corporate Environments: Challenges and Emerging Opportunities.* Walnut Grove, CA: Left Coast Press. 77.

Save the Children. (2013) *Surviving the first day: State of the world's mothers.* Retrieved from: http://www.savethechildren.org/atf/cf/%7B9def2ebe-10ae-432c-9bd0-df91d2eba74a%7D/SOWM-FULL-REPORT_2013.PDF.

Suchman, L. (1995). Making work visible, *Communications of the ACM,* 38(9), 56.

Szymanski, M.H. & Whalen, J. (eds.) (2011). Work practice analysis at Xerox, in Szymanski, M.H., & Whalen, J. (eds.) *Making Work Visible: Ethnographically Grounded Case Studies of Work Practice.* New York: Cambridge University Press.

Tolmie, P. (2011). Uncovering the unremarkable, in Szymanski, M.H., & Whalen, J. (eds.), *Making Work Visible: Ethnographically Grounded Case Studies of Work Practice.* New York: Cambridge University Press.

Widström, A.M. (Producer) (2007). *Breastfeeding: Baby's choice* [DVD]. East Sandwich, MA: Health Education Associates.

Widström, A.M., Lilja, G., Aaltomaa-Michalias, P., Dahllöf, A., Lintula, M., & Nissen, E. (2011). Newborn behaviour to locate the breast when skin-to-skin: A possible method for enabling early self-regulation. *Acta Paediatrica.* 100(1), 79–85.

4

WRITING OF ONE'S OWN CULTURE

An auto-ethnography of home birth midwifery in Ireland

Colm OBoyle

Introduction

This chapter presents my story, an autoethnographic account of how I came to disengage from a woman who had planned to have me as her home birth midwife. This is a personal account where I interrogate my actions and thoughts as research data, and analyse my story and its context. I examine the rhetoric of midwifery professionalism and apply it to my own and the Irish home birth context. The chapter serves three purposes: one, to tell my story; two, to argue that my story, as an exemplar of autoethnography, can be presented as research; and three, to explore the concept of professionalism within midwifery.

Autoethnography: a justification

Before I tell my story, I will give a brief justification of autoethnography as a research methodology. The collectoin titled *Autoethnography* edited by Sikes (2013) gathers together papers by many autoethnographers and those writing about and critiquing autoethnography, I recommend it to those seeking a fuller understanding of the bases and complexities of autoethnography.

Many ethnographies have included an autobiographical or confessional element (Van Maanen 1988). The use of personal and reflexive biographical accounts as research data is then an extension of the ethnographic methodology. The researcher as a visible subject within the field and in the writing is extended to the point where the author's autobiography becomes the research report. The autoethnographer overcomes the conceit of telling someone else's story by admitting theirs is the story they can most legitimately tell. There are two main concerns about autoethnography. The first concern is epistemological, that is, the constitution (and evaluation) of autoethnography as research knowledge.

The other concern is procedural and critiques the ethical use of autobiographic material as research data.

Epistemological issues

The human subject is both constructed by and constructs the world s/he lives in. Writing and storytelling constructs our world. Research, the formal, systematic process of uncovering (or testing) the truth, is a socially constructed attempt to legitimise academic writings above others. Narrative material, literary fiction, journalism and autobiography can, for the researcher, serve as data that can be examined. The application of an analytic process or methodology to that data is what usually constitutes the re-writing as research. That autoethnography begins with, but moves beyond, autobiography is essential. The autoethnographer uses their story to reveal and explore an aspect of the social world they inhabit.

Criteria for evaluation of qualitative inquiry could be applied to autoethnography (Richardson 2000, Tracey 2010, Holman Jones et al. 2013). Evaluative criteria, however, must only be tentative if they are not to become prescriptive and stifling of creativity (Sparkes and Smith 2009). Autoethnographers must steer a course between the evocative, moral and political purposes of autobiography and the legitimising claims of research as rigorous analytical methods. In this autobiography I hope to satisfy both demands.

The story is autobiographical. It is personal, and in it I acknowledge and am reflexive about my subjectivity. I demonstrate a degree of self-searching, and intellectual or moral growth. Linked to that moral awareness, but also to legitimising standards of research practice, I consider the ethical treatment of others. The autobiographical aspects are augmented by more overtly research-based analysis. Within the story I engage with literature in the area and apply a theoretical lens to the analysis of the story. Furthermore, in an element that satisfies both autobiographical and research purposes, my story opens up a socio-political agenda to explore a contested aspect of human social interaction. Finally, any good narrative should be engagingly written; but that judgement ultimately belongs to you, the reader.

Ethical issues

Autoethnography, like ethnography and autobiography is a retrospective endeavour. One cannot really anticipate which social action or interaction will suggest itself as worthy of detailed record and analysis. The autoethnographic researcher cannot anticipate which incidents and people will present interesting issues for sociological examination, but she must consider how to protect such people from any harm inherent in the telling. Again, I recommend Sikes' edited collection *Autoethnography* (2013), particularly volume three 'Ethical concerns around ethnography' in which several authors explore the topic in some depth.

Research ethics requires a degree of anticipatory self-regulation. The requirement of prior informed consent of all participants however is a real sticking point for the autoethnographer. The simple convention of formalised consent-seeking converts a setting from a 'normal' sociological interaction into a somewhat more self-conscious one (see Chapter 1 which mentions the Hawthorn effect, Landsberger 1958). Explicit and formal consent to a 'for the record' interaction changes the social context. There may well be useful insights to be made in such circumstances, but the presentation of an acceptable social face may well obscure the most interesting aspects. Ethnographers must address the consequences of this dilemma of uncovering that which is usually not available for examination.

In order to accommodate autobiographical elements, the autoethnographer must demonstrate conscientious self-regulation which upholds the general principles of ethical behaviour. Physical harm is not the issue in autoethnography but rather the potential for social or reputational harm when the private is made public. Tolich (2010) acknowledges the retrospective nature of autoethnography but recommends that the autoethnographer should still engage with ethics review boards. Wherever possible, anticipatory ethics and process consent should be applied. Where it cannot, Adams (2008) reminds us of the power (and thus the potential for its abuse) that comes with authorship. Tolich, like Ellis (1995) and Medford (2006), reminds us to be wary of publishing that which we would not like written about ourselves. Tolich offers several means by which to ameliorate the potential harm of having one's un-consented story told. He suggests anonymising participants by using pseudonyms and omitting unique identifying features. The use of a fictitious author name or nom de plume can further anonymise those linked to the author of a text. Lastly, retrospective consent may be sought but, as Tolich points out, the inevitably social nature of the relationship between the author and others may make refusal difficult. Ellis (2007) too exhorts us always to recognise and honour our relational responsibilities in autoethnography.

This particular autoethnographic piece contains a further significant ethical concern. That is the inclusion of material about a woman who had been in my care. A health care professional is in a socially responsible and relatively powerful position and so must exercise particular caution in the telling of a client's story. I believe that I have considered this aspect of my relationship with the woman concerned, by retrospectively gaining her explicit consent to report those parts of her story that overlap with my own.

It is not only others who may be vulnerable to harm. Ruth Behar (1996) writes of the vulnerability of the autoethnographer. Even if I write only of myself there may be potential for self-harm, the long-term consequences of which need to be considered. Examination of that which is personally and socially problematic or unacceptable may stigmatise the autoethnographer. Revealing the socially hide-able can be a personally dangerous undertaking. Insights so shared, however, may make further sociological examination possible. I feel vulnerable to reproach from peers about my actions in the story about to be told. I believe though that these feelings of vulnerability and doubt are the emotional expression of my moral dilemma and sense of the (in)justice inherent in the situation (Thompson 2005, McCarthy and Deady 2008).

Ethnography, autoethnography and maternity

Autobiographical accounts of parents', particularly mothers' experiences of birth, are a very common means of making birth visible and accessible to others. These accounts have been used as primary data. Novels and autobiographies of midwifery are also available. Indeed, the popular UK television series *Call the Midwife* was derived from a midwife's autobiography. Ethnographies of maternity settings exist, for example in the work of Hunt and Symonds (1995), Kirkham and Stapleton (2004), Walsh (2006), Frei and Mander (2011), Flacking and Dykes (2013) and OBoyle (2014a) among others, some presented in this volume. I have however been unable to find an autoethnography written by a midwife or obstetrician but the case has been made for the use of autoethnography in nursing (Peterson 2014). My own doctoral work (OBoyle 2009) was an insider ethnography and contained some autobiographical elements but presented largely using interview transcripts as the major data source. The lack of midwifery autoethnography, I believe, reflects the dominance of the scientific paradigm of objective distance which permeates professional discourse in both practice and research. Hierarchies of evidence which privilege the randomised control trial for example, are antipathetic to personal narrative; and so professionals are discouraged from making their stories available to others in 'legitimate' research fora.

Midwifery discourse and the midwifery voice in academic writings could be characterised in two modes. The first engages with positivistic scientific discourse in research papers addressing objective measurement of mortality, morbidity and the like. Other midwifery writings speak of the social context of midwifery and the mother–midwife relationship (Kirkham 2000). Historical perspectives on the nature of midwifery professionalisation, for example, recognise the professional claims and boundary maintenance issues at work within and between medicine and midwifery (Hugman 1991, Witz 1992 and Sandall 1995). Davis-Floyd and Johnson (2006) in the US, Mander and Fleming (2002) and Kirkham (2004) in the UK and Murphy-Lawless (1998) in Ireland, have each acknowledged the socio-political agenda in maternity and midwifery. Acknowledgement of the social and relational approach of midwifery to pregnancy, birth and parenting could form the basis for a political change and a resurgence of midwifery in the organisation of maternity services. While a social or primary care agenda for maternity services in Ireland has been espoused (DoH&C 2001) this would require an enormous structural overhaul. Given the pervasiveness of risk aversion in all its forms, personal, clinical and not least financial, radical political change in Ireland is an uphill struggle.

What can autoethnographic midwifery experience bring to the table? Autoethnography is deeply personal and yet the personal is always socially embedded and to some degree politically freighted. My story tells of how I feel I failed to practise what I 'profess', how I failed to serve, and I analyse how and why this was possible. Autoethnographies of midwifery can reveal to ourselves and to the wider public what it is to be a midwife, to be with, or by contrast in this case, to fail to be with woman at birth.

My story is divided into three parts; in the first I describe my midwifery career and my motivation for undertaking to offer home birth support. The second is my general experience and feeling about being a home birth midwife; its pleasures and demands. These two set the scene for the third part which tells of a particularly distressing incident for me. This last part forms the basis for the subsequent analysis of my response and leads to an exploration of the social context in which home birth midwives operate in Ireland. The social context encompasses midwifery legislation, health service policy, midwifery philosophy and the rhetoric of professionalism and professional jurisdiction. These are each theoretically very complex and yet it is the co-existence of these social elements that makes home birth midwifery in Ireland so challenging and makes my personal story evocative of that challenge. My story is not simply documentary data but enables the theoretical exploration of a particular contemporary social context. It is, I believe, a legitimate piece of sociological research, rigorously presented and ethically considered.

Story part one

I felt, if I was to have any credibility as a researcher of home birth midwifery, I had to do some homebirths myself. I have been a midwife for twenty years and apart from some community midwifery as a student, I have worked as a hospital midwife, mostly in the delivery suite, and latterly as a midwife teacher with very little clinical practice. I have always been attracted by the professional freedom intimated by the term 'autonomous' midwifery practice. My mother had six of my siblings in the bedroom next to mine at home. I believe that for most healthy women, home is likely the best place for them to birth. They are in their own environment, with people they know and trust, and so are likely to come to know their own power in birth. At home, they can avoid the many indignities and interventions which can befall them in an institutional birth setting.

From my years in practice, and as a teacher, I understand that it can be difficult and demoralising to work in a hospital with its routines and protocols, which, with the best will in the world, can stifle women's freedoms and limit the formation of trusting relationships between woman and midwife. Contact between mother and midwife is fragmented and discontinuous. During labour and birth, women and their partners are in an alien environment, often dependent upon a stranger to guide them through the bodily experience of birth and, crucially also, through the complex systems and unfamiliar routines and practices of the hospital. I believed, because of the personal relationship built with women, that birth could be better at home. I believed, because of the relative freedom of independent home birth practice, that I would feel more fulfilled as a home birth midwife than I had been as a hospital midwife or as a midwife teacher. Whilst I enjoyed both these roles very much, I felt a growing disillusionment with the stultifying risk phobia and implacable demands of a resource-strapped 'birth machine'.

Thus informed, or with this frank partiality, I ventured into independent midwifery practice. I felt within myself, and from the response of those midwives who knew and nurtured me, that this step was simultaneously brave and foolhardy; admirable, yet could leave me professionally vulnerable and exposed. I followed several home birth midwives as they worked. One was a colleague I greatly admired for her earthy good sense, for her firm support of women's power to birth, and for her astute awareness of the politics of birthing outside accepted norms. I was moved but unsurprised by the warmth of their relationship with women. I was reminded of the power and normality of labour and birth. I was delighted by the welcome and encouragement offered to me by midwives, women and their families. Before I had properly considered the time and emotional cost of this change of life-course, I was approached by a woman so keen to have a home birth that my gender and my self-perception as a novice did not matter. I recall highlighting and almost apologising to that first couple for my limited home birth experience. I was challenged by their question: 'Do you feel able for this? Because if you are; we are.' I said that I was, and I fervently hoped that I was.

Analysis

In order to progress towards the main thrust of this autoethnography, I will take the opportunity now to break from the story and to explore the main contextual frame within which the story unfolds. This section will focus on the Irish maternity services, particularly the culture and context of home birth midwifery practice in Ireland. My behaviour can, I hope, be understood in that context. My purpose is to use my story to explore and challenge to the maternity service culture in Ireland.

I have been unable to avoid allowing something of my partiality for home birth as an alternative to hospital birth to come to the fore. To me home birth seems a good choice for most women but also for midwifery autonomy. I will not explore this idea further or more explicitly in this analysis. Other writers have done so from both women's (notably Edwards 2005, Cheyney 2011) and midwives' perspectives (particularly Davis-Floyd and Johnson 2006, Vedam et al. 2009). I have to acknowledge however my own enthusiasm for both women's birthing autonomy and a midwife's ability, indeed duty as professional servant (Cronk 2000), to facilitate it. My story then is open about my subjectivity and situatedness. This is fitting for an ethnographer as such openness gives narrative research texts what Sandra Harding (1996) called 'strong objectivity'.

The structure of the health service in the Republic of Ireland is not the same as in Great Britain and Northern Ireland. Ireland gained independence from Britain in 1926, well before the inauguration of the National Health Service in Britain. Ireland has had a mixed public and private health service ever since. A medical card system provides free care for those of limited means and it was only as late as the 1990s that maternity care became free for all. Home birth, as in most other Western countries, was discouraged from the mid-twentieth century. The services of district or community midwives became redundant and birth and midwifery practice became almost exclusively hospital based. Unlike the UK therefore, Ireland has no national community midwifery service to provide postnatal care, and supports very few home births (fewer than 0.5 per cent since the 1980s, Economic and Social Research Institute 2013). There have been a few attempts to expand birth choices for women with isolated schemes for home birth in Cork, Kerry, Waterford and a small area in part of south Dublin, initiated as pilot schemes in the late 1990s. Two midwifery led units were opened in the north east in the early 2000s and several hospitals, particularly in Dublin, have begun systems to provide midwifery support for early postnatal transfer home (within 12 hours). Taken together, this all sounds quite positive for women's birth choices, but these small schemes are inadequate in capacity and geographically unevenly distributed. This leaves Irish women, even those considered to be low risk and suitable for midwifery models of care, in something of a postcode lottery. Furthermore, attempts by women to demand that the Health Service Executive (HSE) provide them with the choice of home birth have been rebutted. The Supreme Court in 2003 ruled that the HSE could not be obliged to provide home birth. In 2013, a woman who had found a midwife who would be willing to attend her for a home birth after a previous caesarean section, was told by the High Court that the HSE again could not be obliged to provide a care package it felt had a significant clinical risk. That woman subsequently went to Northern Ireland for her birth.

It can be seen then that in Ireland hospital midwifery is the norm and there are very few opportunities for midwifery-led care. There are however still a handful of (less than twenty) midwives who offer home birth beyond the few hospital outreach DOMINO and home birth schemes mentioned. The 'national' home birth scheme that depends on these few midwives will be discussed in the next section but prior to this a last aspect of midwifery practice in Ireland that is distinctly different from the UK needs to be mentioned.

Midwifery supervision is a statutory mechanism in the UK for the support and maintenance of good-quality professional midwifery services to the public. Each midwife has a named supervisor who ensures that the midwife maintains their competence. Each midwife, perhaps especially those in more isolated practice, such as independent midwives, has access to a senior professional colleague who has some power to support midwives to provide for women's choice and birthing autonomy. If a woman were to decline midwifery advice in some regard, the midwife could call upon her supervisor to facilitate the woman's informed choice regarding her pregnancy, birth and maternity care. In the UK, unlike Ireland, woman's birth choices are systematically supported and enabled rather than declined or withheld. The midwifery philosophy of being 'with woman' is upheld in the UK by a combination of the NHS provision of birth choices and professional midwifery structures of supervision. As will be demonstrated, these mechanisms are not available to Irish home birth midwives.

Story part two

I have spoken a little about the demands of hospital midwifery. There is fragmentation of the integrity of pregnancy and birth into wards and hospital departments dedicated to pregnancy, birth or postnatal care. There are long days, shift work, and regular rotation to night duty. There is less autonomy of practice within the hierarchy of hospital and a greater subservience of midwifery to obstetrics, than I had anticipated at the outset of my career.

The demands of independent home birth midwifery are altogether different. I can take on as few or as many women as I wish. I can accept or turn down cases on grounds of both geographical convenience and my own professional judgement about suitability for home delivery. I can decline to take on people due to subtleties of personality mismatch. The hospital midwife has no such luxury. A good working relationship between the lone midwifery practitioner and the home birth woman is so essential that the lack of 'click', or presence of strain in the relationship, even in the earliest interaction, can legitimise the dissolution of negotiations to contract to each other. It took me some time to fully realise the mutuality of the trusting relationship between mother and midwife. Yes, she must trust that I will be supportive of her and knowledgeable about birth; but I must also trust that she will recognise that there may come a point where my expertise might, and indeed from my perspective must, take precedence in decisions about how to 'manage' certain deviations from broad healthy 'norms'.

I come to know the woman and her family better in the months of her pregnancy. This is a periodic relationship, built over several one-hour or longer meetings in her home; more often than not with her partner and sometimes children. We negotiate appointment times that are convenient to us both and I get to know her home and the route to it from mine.

Approaching a woman's expected date of birth, we discuss how she will identify the early stages of labour and her arrangements for contacting me. I am 'on call' 24 hours a day, from 37 weeks of pregnancy up until 42 weeks, at which time my contract with the HSE says I may no longer attend for home birth. Being available for these five weeks is quite restrictive to my social freedoms. I cannot stray too far away or enjoy alcohol as freely, as it would disable my ability to be fully present to her. My birthing equipment must always be at the ready and I have a taxi company on speed dial. I have to be able to drop, renegotiate or find alternative provision for my social life and teaching responsibilities. Overall however I am in the relatively privileged position of having a flexible and tolerant partner and no one immediately dependent upon me.

While being on call is something of a burden, working in isolation is, for me, an even bigger one. The wide geographical dispersion of the small number of self-employed midwives, as well as variation in workload and other commitments, seems not to facilitate working partnerships. In hospital practice I could easily consult with colleagues; in home birth practice I can telephone one or two other home birth midwives, but the awareness that professionally the buck stops with me, is somehow more acute.

When I am in bed and know that any one of several women may go into labour overnight, I find that I do not sleep soundly. I go through checklists in my head as I try to go to sleep. My dreams can be more than usually filled with birth imagery and symbols. I get a little fixated with the whereabouts of my phone, whether it is charged, and worry that the 'on silent' button has accidentally been pressed. Even though my equipment is prepared, the possibility of traffic jams or weather events can introduce tension. If I go for a swim I feel I need to text to let mothers know I will be incommunicado even if only for that short time. I, like many of the women I attend, can hardly wait for the waiting to be over. Like the woman herself, I look forward to the excitement and joy of birth. I am aware of, and am prepared for but try not to dwell on, the negative possibilities. In truth it is not only the woman who is expectant but the midwife also; expectant of a normal healthy birth and baby, but alert for signs otherwise.

The phone call comes, and the decision has to be made whether to go to her this instant or to leave her to cope with early labour as we have discussed. This is a tricky judgement over the telephone, even for a midwife. How does she sound emotionally, and physically? How frequent are the contractions? How long and strong and since when? Have the waters gone? Is the baby moving? Can I hear her speaking easily through a contraction or stopping because it is so intense? Can I hear a catch in her breath that might suggest she is nearly ready to push? Am I, as has happened, speaking instead to a husband because his wife has locked herself in the toilet and 'she is making strange and grunting noises'? Do I need to call an ambulance to get there faster than me? Whichever end of the continuum of urgency, there is a sense of relief that at last, things are under way. My midwifery skills and experience is being called upon. I am doing my job rather than just waiting to do my job.

I have been known to say, 'babies all come out the same way' and while to some extent that is true, every birth is different. Some are fast and urgent, some are long and slow. Either can be a good and positive experience or a negative and long-remembered experience for the mother. I get great satisfaction from feeling that my presence, my relationship with the birthing woman, can be the catalyst for the former and a defence against the latter. Perhaps I over inflate my importance but women's own stories about other midwives and other births, sustain my belief in the relevance of the mother–midwife relationship to women's perception of the quality of their birth.

To be with a woman, a couple as they become parents, as they meet their offspring for the very first time, whatever the mode of birth, is thrilling. It is a privilege to share in the final resolution of the anticipation of pregnancy. It is, to me still, an awe-inspiring biological, undeniably earthy process.

The birth attendant, I believe, because it is true for me, cannot but be moved by this transformation. Every birth brings, indeed perhaps demands, an existential realisation of and reflection on the miracle of life, death, and the human need for meaning.

I come home from a birth, often many hours after I have dropped everything at work, or climbed out of bed in the small hours of the morning, and I am buzzing with endorphins; I'm just dying to tell, even those who perhaps could hardly care, all about it. I want to spread the love, joy and good news and report 'all is well, a grand big healthy girl, nine pounds, breastfeeding beautifully, with mum and dad tired but delighted'. Not for me, not for one moment, a pessimistic nod to global overcrowding, declining living standards for future generations, or the possibilities of poverty, pestilence and war. New life, new opportunities, optimism and hope pervade.

Analysis

Again, I take a moment from the story to explore how the HSE home birth scheme simultaneously enables and yet, given changes in the legislative environment of professional health practice in Europe, also severely constrains midwifery support of home birth in Ireland.

A health professional must have clinical indemnity insurance. This requirement is contained within EU directive 2011/24/EU (European Parliament and Council 2011) and is enshrined in the Nurses and Midwives Act (Government of Ireland 2011) which explicitly requires midwifery indemnification for birth attendance. This requirement is fulfilled for hospital midwives through the state-sponsored clinical indemnity scheme (State Claims Agency 2012a, 2012b).

Self-employed midwives had trade union insurance for their practice but it was removed in 2007. In 2008, the HSE inaugurated a mechanism for the indemnification of self-employed community midwives (SECMs). They were offered a memorandum of understanding (MOU) that enabled indemnified midwifery attendance to very low risk women only. While welcomed as a means to allow home birth midwifery to continue, this arrangement prevents the self-employed midwife attending women with even minor or potential complications. Previously, midwives had been able to individually assess and attend women who were fully informed of the possible additional risks of home birth. The National Institute for Health and Care Excellence (NICE) guidelines on place of birth (NICE 2014 section 1.1.10) suggests individual assessment of a number of potentially complicating conditions. The guidelines have largely been adopted by the HSE, but the HSE has however placed the responsibility for individual assessment of these conditions on to obstetricians only and not the midwives who had heretofore advised and, on occasion, attended those women.

Obstetricians have been reluctant to accept the implied responsibility for sanctioning home birth overseen by a midwife not within their immediate sphere of influence. This has left midwives without sanction to attend and thus left women without access to a home birth.

That there is any mechanism for the provision of indemnified home birth is to be celebrated. Many European countries struggle with the new directive due either to reluctance of private insurance companies to provide such cover or the prohibitive costs to independent midwifery practitioners (Abbott 2007, RCM and NMC 2011). The HSE acknowledges that their 'national home birth scheme' does not provide for equity or full availability, even for those fully eligible (HSE 2008 p. 8). As the only means by which a home birth midwife may now legally practise it actually represents a removal of choice to many women. From a midwife perspective, the MOU which ties indemnification to highly restricted 'suitability criteria', also represents a significant diminution of professional autonomy.

The HSE, in its attempt to avoid liability, contracts to serve the lowest risk women only. Significantly, however, it is the individual midwife who must enforce the contract by personally declining or withdrawing from the woman's care. The woman seeking home birth is asked to confirm she will transfer to hospital care if she develops any risk factor during pregnancy or labour. What is of concern to an SECM is that a woman may decline to transfer to hospital in these cases. The midwife is then exposed to attending a woman outside the terms of the HSE scheme. Outside of the scheme the midwife is uninsured and, uninsured, the midwife is outside the law. The SECMs have raised these concerns with the HSE, however, and their appeals for clear and suitable guidance have not, yet, been met.

Story part three

> I was asked to be the midwife for Anna (pseudonym) who is expecting her first baby. I met with her and her partner Paul (pseudonym). She was well and healthy with no contraindications for home birth and they both seemed very committed to a home birth and to avoiding interventions. I

agreed to take her on and she applied to the HSE for a home birth. All went well during the pregnancy but as her expected date of birth approached she became concerned that the terms of the home birth scheme, which she had signed her agreement to, indicated that I could not attend her after 42 weeks gestation. She approached the hospital in which she was booked and negotiated a recalculation of her due date but as even that deadline approached she became increasingly agitated by the limits of the scheme and the hospital consultant's insistence that she come to hospital for induction of labour. She was well informed and could cite the evidence of the risks associated with prolonged pregnancy. She preferred to avoid intervention. The hospital consultant proposed alternate day monitoring of the baby to postpone unwanted induction, but would not sanction home birth past 42 weeks. Her reported relationship with the hospital and her perception of their inflexibility led me to believe that if some accommodation were not made, she might withdraw from professional contact altogether and choose to birth alone. I contacted the HSE to outline my concern and to offer to attend beyond the terms of the home birth scheme. I asked if they would enable me to do so by sanctioning my attendance outside the scheme and continuing to professionally indemnify me. They would not.

I was acutely uncomfortable with the prospect of withdrawing my support and explicitly refusing to attend her in birth after 42 weeks. This was a woman I had grown to know well and who I knew was resolute in her belief in her ability to birth outside of hospital. I felt I was being forced, by the terms of the contract with the HSE, to abandon this woman. The emotional cost to Anna and to me seemed of no concern to the HSE. The default response appeared to be risk avoidance rather than risk management. I felt that the HSE representative was avoiding setting a precedent for midwifery attendance outside the strictest terms of the scheme. Higher clinical risks are clearly not within the scope of the scheme. Whatever emotional discomfort that brings to the woman or the midwife in such a case, the service limits are clear. I felt professionally conflicted.

It seemed clear to me from both the HSE and my regulatory body (the Nursing and Midwifery Board of Ireland, NMBI) that I should signal that hospital birth was the only option now being offered to Anna. It was clear to me that if I facilitated a home birth outside the scheme, any claim for professional compensation would have to be met entirely from my own financial resources. Furthermore I felt acutely vulnerable that signalling any willingness to facilitate an out-of-hospital birth would have to bear close inspection by both the HSE and the NMBI. It was clear that the HSE and the NMBI felt that Anna's choice about where to birth was still hers to make. I was led to doubt whether my professional reputation in contractual relationship with the HSE and the professional requirement for indemnification would support attendance at Anna's birth. I said to Anna that although I believe in informed birth choice and 'being with woman', I felt I could not jeopardise my professional registration, reputation and livelihood. Anna and Paul said they understood, sympathised and that they would not test my resolve by calling me in an 'emergency'; a circumstance in which I believe they knew I could not and would not abandon them. Nonetheless, I feel that I, like the HSE and NMBI, passed the consequences of my unwillingness to accommodate Anna's choices back to her. I, like them, passed rather than accepted the buck.

The saddest part of this whole story is yet to be told. Anna broke off contact with the hospital, and refused to respond to calls from the HSE. Anna left her Dublin home and went to stay elsewhere. This, I understood, was in some part due to uncertainty about whether she might be forced to go to hospital. Afterwards Anna confirmed this was an issue, but that she had wanted to go into labour where she felt close to the supports of her family. Anna said she thought she would present herself to hospital well advanced in labour in the hope of avoiding interventions. In truth, I don't know if all had gone well that she would have gone to hospital. In any event, as she told me afterwards, Anna felt that the baby stopped moving and that Paul could no longer hear the fetal heart with his ear to her abdomen. They went to a local hospital and an ultrasound scan there confirmed that the baby had died. She birthed her dead baby in that hospital.

I will not try to pretend to understand or begin to describe how Anna and Paul felt and feel about that turn of events and how it colours their view of the preceding experiences and decisions. I can describe my own feelings. I am ashamed to say that my first conscious reaction after the shock and sadness at hearing the news, was a sense of gratitude that I had distanced myself, even though I had felt, and still feel ashamed for doing so. If I had been resolute and stood by her and my claimed philosophy of being 'with woman' I might have spotted signs that the baby was in trouble. In this knowledge, Anna might well have accepted that hospital was now clearly an appropriate choice, the better alternative. I must bear that possibility, that lost opportunity, and accept the consequences of my part in the scenario. Had I stayed with Anna, 'with woman' however, and if the baby had still died, then I, as the autonomous clinician, one who had clearly transgressed the professionally acceptable boundaries of an agreed contract and of indemnified practice, would clearly bear the greater burden of blame. I have outlined and can retrace my decisions and my many motivations and query the wisdom of my emotional involvement before during and after this incident, but I have no doubt that had the baby died, the HSE and the NMBI would have judged me harshly. Even if the baby had lived and the home birth had been a success, my professionalism would have come under close scrutiny and perhaps reproach. My first reaction then was one of relief from that possibility. My second was one of guilt for having abandoned Anna, but that deed was done, the consequences, the shame and culpability, should be no greater. I had let her down, I had let myself down and I had, perhaps in the eyes of some my peers, let my profession down.

No one wanted this baby to die. All of us involved probably recognise that we could have acted differently. I know Anna feels that the anticipation of running out of time and the close monitoring of the baby was stressful to her. She feels that together these inhibited her going into easy spontaneous labour and that together these stressors killed her baby. That health care professionals do not accept stress as a mechanism for cause of death, contributes to Anna's anger and her grief. I met with Anna some weeks afterwards to talk with her about her, their, and my own feelings around the last days of the pregnancy and the loss of their baby. I asked them about their access to support, their relationship and their plans for future babies. I wasn't looking for forgiveness for my part in our story, but I wanted to share my perspective with them. Even in their grief they allowed me that, and I believe they understood.

Anna has since had another baby. She wanted a home birth again but was not facilitated by the HSE home birth scheme to plan one. Her history placed her beyond their suitability criteria. The baby was born in hospital and breastfed. Mother, father and baby (now almost two years old) are well.

Analysis

Thus far in the analytic sections the differences between the Irish and UK maternity service contexts have been discussed. So too has the unique arrangement for a 'national' home birth service which relies upon a small number of self-employed community midwives whose autonomy is restricted by the tying their indemnification to a narrow set of suitability criteria. The last part of my story tells of my collusion with a 'service' which fails to serve so many women who would like, but cannot access, midwifery attendance at home.

My understanding of what happened can be explained in terms of opposing conceptions of professionalism and professionalisation. Friedson (2001) argues that the utility of professional expertise in service of society justifies their power to self-regulate. Friedson describes professional autonomy as a third and distinct mode of social governance; different from both bureaucratic governmental forces and market forces. Professionalism describes the inherent qualities of service, but professionalisation is the collective means by which occupations sustain the elevated status of profession. Occupational boundary maintenance and concern for continuing recognition, legitimacy and status for the midwifery profession can undermine its service philosophy (OBoyle 2014b).

Professional knowledge and skills have a recognised place in childbirth. The woman who has engaged a birth attendant, has acknowledged their skills, knowledge and experience with regard to the process birth and the potential for its management. The context of the home as a place of birth is very different from hospital where it can be assumed that 'doctor knows best'. Expressions of power and relationship are different in the home where the woman's power and autonomy are an explicitly validated and normalised professional status. Kirkham (2000), Lundgren and Berg (2007) and McCourt and Stevens (2008) highlight the significance of the mother–midwife relationship in supporting positive, autonomous birthing. Calvert (2002) and Mander (2001) have critiqued the distancing effect of a formal professional–client relationship which diminishes the relationship and demotes its importance as secondary to professional authority. Billie Hunter, in particular, writes about the emotion work of midwifery arising from its highly relational nature (Hunter 2004, Hunter et al. 2008, Hunter and Deery 2008).

In my story, I demoted the relationship and the philosophy of 'being with', to the limited definition of a professional as one who is obedient to the law and compliant to the restrictive guidelines of the HSE. I failed in my professional service by a greater concern for professionalisation, the maintenance of my professional status. I upheld the boundaries set upon or by my profession. I attempted to maintain my professional status by privileging the requirement for indemnification. I accepted the limitations on my insurance and therefore on my practice contracted with the HSE. I believed that in Ireland, to remain with Anna outside the HSE contracted scheme would be frowned upon not only by the HSE but also by my profession because it would have left me on the wrong side of the law, that is, without indemnity. I knew that the HSE had already had Supreme (2003) and High Court (2013) approval for its withholding of home birth choice from women except on the HSE's own terms. Taken together, any decision to remain with Anna would be taken as flouting all of these professionally supported restrictions on my continued attendance.

By holding to the contracted limits to my attendance however, I behaved in a way that was inconsistent with my philosophy of being with woman. I colluded in the removal of her choice of professionally attended birth at home and in the attempt to make her conform to a narrow judgement as to the (ab)normality and appropriate risk management of her birth. The outcome, a baby born dead in hospital, might have been the same, or it might not. Tragic as the outcome was and might still have been had I stayed, the fact that I chose to preserve my professional status before my 'being with' philosophy and my personal relationship with her is a disappointment to me. I feel I have failed to behave morally.

I believe in the primacy of the professional requirement to serve women's birthing autonomy. That is the basis of the mother–midwife relationship. Social and political circumstances in Ireland currently obstruct that relationship. The HSE's lack of support for continued indemnified midwifery attendance in changed circumstances, or in the face of a woman's decision to remain at home despite developing contraindications, left me and leaves other home birth midwives professionally exposed. My story reveals how acutely distressing the demands of professionalism can be in the context of home birth midwifery in contemporary Ireland. That home birth midwives feel under threat from their own profession is supported by their anticipation of harsh critique in Ireland (OBoyle 2013). In broader international and interdisciplinary contexts, Wagner (2007) goes as far as to describe professional control of their non-normative members as akin to a witch hunt.

Davis-Floyd however in her book *Mainstreaming Midwives* (2006) describes how the existence of some midwives who push, or simply reject, the boundaries of acceptable professional practice, maximise the rhetorical, social and practical space for the greater number of other, less radical, midwives. Perhaps home birth midwives in Ireland perform something of the same function. I would like to add my story to the canon that argues for a radical reconsideration of the values that underpin Irish maternity services. The argument, in Ireland, that women's safety lies at the centre of the many restrictions to midwifery autonomy is, I believe, false. My story is just one that demonstrates how current provision is failing not only women but also the midwives who would support them.

Discussion

This chapter has presented a personal story that moves beyond simple first-person narrative or autobiography. The personal moral dilemma that lies at the heart of the story has been explored by the protagonist as a self-aware subject situated in a particular social context. The story then has become more than simple data by the explication of context and by the application of an analytical framing of the personal experience as an exemplar of a contested socio-political issue.

Narratives can be explored by outsiders in many ways but the insider or emic perspective can most easily be accessed, presented and analysed by the reflective subject. That is the essence of autoethnography, which acknowledges the subjectivity not only of social actors but also of those who re-present human behaviour and narrative as research. The telling and retelling of stories serve those who tell and those who listen. Researchers and academics emphasise the analytic and theoretic elements of their narrative product and legitimise their endeavours with talk of ethical probity. The autoethnographer is subjectively engaged and must convince her readers that her autobiography can legitimately claim the name research. Any innovation must present its case for legitimacy and claim its place amongst the established canon. Tolich (2010) argues that autoethnography has succeeded to some extent in claiming its place as an established research methodology. I believe however that autoethnographers, for the time being at least, must still argue the case for recognition of their analytic narrative product as research.

The retrospective nature of autobiographic narratives make prior research community approval almost impossible to obtain. The introduction of this chapter outlined the ethical implications of this reality. The explicit consideration and application of ethical principles in the temporal space between unplanned experience, and the analysis and subsequent presentation of the experience, can alleviate almost all harm and potential for harm to those written into the narrative. This post-hoc arrangement for the demonstration of ethical conduct has yet to find a secure place in research academe where ethical approval is conceptualised as a pre-research process. A further specific ethical concern in this case was the inclusion of material, both clinical and personal, about someone to whom I had privileged professional access. The retrospective use of clinical case material in other research contexts has however been legitimised and mechanisms for its use accommodated.

I have presented an analysis of my feelings of regret at abandoning the philosophical principle of 'being with' woman (a professional attribute of service) in favour of protecting my status as an indemnified and thus 'legitimate' professional. That I, a midwife in Ireland, find myself torn between these choices, reveals a contested aspect of social interaction (Thompson 2005) beyond the already well-documented limitations to women's birth choices in Ireland (Devane 2007). Professional indemnification and its arrangements are the result of a neoliberal commodification of professional service within a blame and compensation culture which is becoming increasingly prevalent in the West. Actuarial concern for the costs and financial risk associated with malpractice and compensation, which have come to pervade health and maternity care, are, I believe, partly bureaucratic but essentially market-driven rather than properly professional.

Insofar as the midwifery profession in Ireland chooses to accept and privilege market-driven restrictions on their service, we privilege the demands of professional status above our own autonomy and women's birthing autonomy. There is no collective midwifery voice in Ireland which might contest such a limited conceptualisation of what it is to be professional. This means that individual practitioners are placed in the invidious position of choosing between the privileges of their title and their relationship with the birthing woman. I believe that my individual experience reveals and speaks to a contested and yet underexplored social and political agenda in Ireland and perhaps elsewhere. What is it to be a professional? What is it to be a midwife? And what, if anything, do Irish midwives want to do about the peculiar regulatory context in which contemporary Irish home birth midwives work?

I leave you with a final question that is at the very heart of any evaluation or critique of qualitative research; has this autoethnography engaged you? I have told my story, make of it what you will.

References

Abbott, L (2007). Insuring independent midwives. *RCM Midwives: The Official Journal of the Royal College of Midwives* 10.8 (discussion), 393.

Adams, TE (2008) A review of narrative ethics. *Qualitative Inquiry* 14(2) 175–194.

Behar, R (1996) *The Vulnerable Observer*, Boston, MA: Beacon Press.

Calvert, S (2002) Being with women: The midwife–woman relationship. In Mander, R and Fleming, V (eds) *Failure to Progress: The Contraction of the Midwifery Profession*. London: Routledge.

Cheyney, M (ed.) (2011). *Born at Home, The Biological, Cultural and Political Dimensions of Maternity Care in the United States*. Studies in Contemporary Social Issues. Belmont CA : Wadsworth.

Cronk, M (2000). The midwife: A professional servant? In M Kirkham (ed.), *The Midwife–Mother Relationship*. London: Macmillan.

Davis-Floyd, R, and Johnson, CB (eds) (2006) *Mainstreaming Midwives: The Politics of Change*. New York: Routledge.

Department of Health and Children (2001) *Primary Care: A New Direction*. Dublin: The Stationery Office.

Devane, D (2007). Normal birth in Ireland. *AIMS Journal (Association for Improvements in the Maternity Services UK)*, 19(2), 20–21.

Economic and Social Research Institute, Health Research and Information Division (ESRI 2012) *Perinatal Statistics Report 2011*, Dublin. http://www.esri.ie/UserFiles/publications/SUSTAT46.pdf. Accessed on 20 October 2013.

Edwards, NP (2005) *Birthing Autonomy: Women's Experiences of Planning Home Births*, London: Routledge.

Ellis C (1995) Emotional and ethical quagmires in returning to the field. *Journal of Contemporary Ethnography* 24, 711–713.

Ellis C (2007) Telling secrets, revealing lives: relational ethics in research with intimate others. *Qualitative Inquiry* 13(1) 3–29.

European Parliament and Council (2011) Directive 2011/24/EU: on the application of patients' rights in cross-border healthcare. *Official Journal of the European Union* http://eur-lex.europa.eu/legal-content/EN/TXT/?uri=uriserv:OJ.L_.2011.088.01.0045.01. ENG Accessed on 8 October 2014.

Flacking R, and Dykes F (2013) 'Being in a womb' or 'playing musical chairs': the impact of place and space on infant feeding in NICUs. *BMC Pregnancy and Childbirth* 13: 179 http://www.biomedcentral.com/content/pdf/1471-2393-13-179.pdf

Frei, IA, and Mander, R (2011) The relationship between first-time mothers and care providers in the early postnatal phase: an ethnographic study in a Swiss postnatal unit. *Midwifery* 27 (5) 716–722.

Friedson, E (2001). *Professionalism: The Third Logic*. Chicago, IL: University of Chicago Press.

Government of Ireland (2011) Nurses and Midwives Act. Dublin: The Stationery Office.

Harding, S (1996) Feminism, science, and the anti-establishment critiques. In Garry, A and Pearsall, M (eds) *Women, Knowledge, and Reality: Explorations in Feminist Philosophy*. New York: Routledge.

Health Service Executive (HSE). (2008). *Delivery on Choice: Homebirth Options for Women in Ireland*. Domiciliary Birth Implementation Group Report. Dublin: HSE.

High Court (2013) EIHC 383, *Teehan* v. *Health Service Executive* http://www.bailii.org/ie/cases/IEHC/2013/H383.html Accessed on 20 September 2013.

Holman Jones S, Adams T, and Ellis C (eds) (2013). *Handbook of Autoethnography*. Walnut Grove, CA: Left Coast Press.

Hugman, R (1991) *Power in Caring Professions*. London: Palgrave Macmillan.

Hunt, S, and Symonds, A (1995) *The Social Meaning of Midwifery*. Basingstoke: Macmillan.

Hunter, B (2004) Conflicting ideologies as a source of emotion work in midwifery. *Midwifery*, 20, 261–272.

Hunter, B, and Deery, R (eds) (2008) *Emotions in Midwifery and Reproduction.* London: Palgrave Macmillan.

Hunter, B, Berg, M, Lundgren, I, Olafdottir, OA, and Kirkham, M (2008) Relationships: The hidden threads in the tapestry of maternity care. *Midwifery* 24, 132–137.

Kirkham, M (2000) How can we relate? In Kirkham, M (ed.) *The Midwife–Mother Relationship.* London: Macmillan.

Kirkham, M, and Stapleton, H (2004) The culture of the maternity services. In Kirkham, M (ed.) *Informed Choice in Maternity Care.* Basingstoke: Palgrave Macmillan.

Landsberger, HA (1958). *Hawthorne Revisited.* Ithaca, NY: Cornell University Press.

Lundgren, I, and Berg, M (2007) Central concepts in the midwife–woman relationship *Scandinavian Journal of Caring Sciences*, 21, 220–228.

Mander, R (2001) *Supportive Care and Midwifery.* Oxford: Blackwell Science.

Mander, R, and Fleming, V (2002) *Failure to Progress: The Contraction of the Midwifery Profession.* Philadelphia, PA: Psychology Press,

McCarthy, J, and Deady, R (2008). Moral distress reconsidered. *Nursing Ethics*, 15, 254–262.

McCourt, C, and Stevens, T (2008) Relationship and reciprocity in caseload midwifery In Hunter, B and Deery, R (eds.) *Emotions in Midwifery and Reproduction.* London: Palgrave Macmillan.

Medford K (2006) Caught with fake ID: Ethical questions about slippage in autoethnography. *Qualitative Inquiry* 12, 853–864.

Murphy-Lawless, J (1998). *Reading Birth and Death: A History of Obstetric Thinking.* Cork: Cork University Press.

National Institute for Health and Care Excellence (NICE). (2014). Intrapartum Care CG 190 https://www.nice.org.uk/guidance/cg190/chapter/recommendations Accessed on 19 December 2014.

OBoyle, C (2009) An ethnography of independent midwifery in Ireland. Unpublished PhD Thesis, Trinity College Dublin.

OBoyle, C (2013) 'Just waiting to be hauled over the coals': Home birth midwifery in Ireland. *Midwifery*, 29 (8), 988–995.

OBoyle, C (2014a) 'Being with' while retaining and asserting professional midwifery power and authority in home birth. *Journal of Organisational Ethnography* 3 (2) 204–223.

OBoyle, C (2014b). The context and consequences of professional indemnification of home birth midwifery in Ireland. *International Journal of Childbirth*, 4(1), 39–54.

Peterson, AL (2014) A case for the use of autoethnography in nursing research. *Journal of Advanced Nursing.* http://onlinelibrary.wiley.com/doi/10.1111/jan.12501/pdf

Richardson, L (2000) Evaluating ethnography. *Qualitative Inquiry* 6 (2) 253–255.

Royal College of Midwives and Nursing and Midwifery Council (RCM & NMC). (2011). *The Feasibility and Insurability of Independent Midwifery in England.* London: Flaxman Partners, RCM.

Sandall, J (1995). Choice, continuity and control: changing midwifery, towards a sociological perspective. *Midwifery*, 11, 201–209.

Sikes, P (ed.) (2013) *Autoethnography.* London: Sage Publications.

Sparkes AC, and Smith B (2009) Judging the quality of qualitative inquiry: criteriology and relativism in action. *Psychology of Sport and Exercise* 10, 491–497.

State Claims Agency. (2012a). Clinical Indemnity Scheme. http://www.stateclaims.ie/ClinicalIndemnityScheme/introduction.html Accessed 21 November 2012.

State Claims Agency. (2012b). Self Employed Community Midwives. http://www.stateclaims.ie/ClinicalIndemnityScheme/publications/2010/SECMSept2010.pdf Accessed 21 November 2012.

Supreme Court (2003) IESC 56 *O'Brien v. South Western Area Health Board, Brannick v East Coast Area HealthBoard, Clarke - South Western Area Health Board, Lockhart v South Western Area Health Board.* http://www.supremecourt.ie/Judgments.nsf/1b0757edc3 71032e802572ea0061450e/c8e6d502f9c0512d80256def00518e49?OpenDocument Accessed on 20 September 2013.

Thompson, F (2005). The emotional impact on mothers and midwives of conflict between workplace and personal/professional ethics. *Australian Midwifery Journal*, 18(3), 17–21.

Tolich, M (2010). A critique of current practice: Ten foundational guideleines for autoethnographers. *Qualitative Health Research*, 20(12), 1599–1610.

Tracey, SJ (2010) Qualitative quality: eight 'big-tent' criteria for excellent qualitative research. *Qualitative Inquiry* 16 (10) 837–851.

Van Maanen, J (1988) *Tales of the Field: On Writing Ethnography*, Chicago, IL: University of Chicago Press.

Vedam, S, Stoll, K, White, S, Aaker, J, and Schummers, L (2009). Nurse-midwives' experiences with planned home birth: impact on attitudes and practice. *Birth*, 36(4), 274–282.

Wagner, M (2007) Birth and power. In Savage, W (ed.) *Birth and Power: A Savage Enquiry Revisited.* London: Middlesex University Press.

Walsh, D (2006) Subverting assembly-line birth: Childbirth in a free-standing birth centre. *Social Science & Medicine* 62(6), 1330–1340.

Witz, A (1992) *Professions and Patriarchy.* London: Routledge.

5

A MIRROR ON PRACTICE

Using ethnography to identify and facilitate best practice in maternity and child health care

Virginia Schmied, Elaine Burns and
Hannah Dahlen

Introduction

Research in the fields of implementation science and knowledge translation reports resistance to policy and practice change and emphasises the need for multidisciplinary approaches to address the challenges of implementing international evidence or best practice principles into practice. In our research into maternity and child health care we have employed ethnographic methods, particularly observations of midwifery and child and family health (CFH) nursing practice, to understand how organisational culture and individual professional practice influence experiences and outcomes of the women and families who use maternity and CFH health services in New South Wales, Australia.

In this chapter we draw on three of our studies to examine the implementation of evidence-based practice in midwifery and also child and family health nursing services. These three studies examined: 1) the implementation of routine psychosocial assessment and depression screening in the perinatal period (Rollans, Schmied, Kemp, & Meade, 2013a, 2013b, 2013c); 2) the facilitators and barriers to physiological birth positioning (Dahlen et al., 2010; Priddis, Dahlen, & Schmied, 2011, 2012) and 3) the implementation of principles and strategies to support the initiation and establishment of breastfeeding (Burns, Fenwick, Sheehan, & Schmied, 2013; Burns, Schmied, Fenwick, & Sheehan, 2012). In undertaking these studies, each in a different hospital and community setting, we were struck by the similarities across the findings, particularly in relation to the approach to practice taken by individual midwives and nurses, as well as the nature of the organisational culture and the structural barriers to evidence-based practice.

An ethnographic approach has allowed us to take a 'micro-perspective' or a close-up view of 'the Institution' and how it works, including an understanding of the cultures and how players act and feel in this context, and where the contradictions and areas of social conflict lie. In these studies we noticed a difference between what midwives and nurses say they do, or what they recognise as best practice, and what they actually do when observed in the practice setting. Ethnographic methods also allowed us to observe what professionals do in practice and to explore the impact of the environment on practice. In this chapter, we re-examine our published findings by drawing on concepts from Michel Foucault to critically examine how power is distributed and exercised and the way in which the language and practices of health professionals and organisational culture influence the implementation of evidence-based policies and best-practice guidelines.

Evidence-based practice and knowledge translation: contemporary critique

Evidence-based practice is defined as "the conscientious, explicit and judicious use of current best evidence in making decisions about the care of the individual patient. It means integrating individual clinical expertise with the best available external clinical evidence from systematic research" (Sackett, Rosenberg, Gray, Muir Haynes, & Richardson, 1996, p. 71). Translating research into practice in the health care environment involves integrating the best available evidence into established routines, procedures and into health practitioner communication. However, significant problems have been identified when translating evidence into practice. The problem of getting evidence into practice has been identified previously as an innovation gap (i.e. a lack of high-quality research evidence), but after many years of research activity it is now recognised that there are areas where robust research evidence exists, and yet health professionals fail to use this evidence in practice (Greenhalgh, Robert, Macfarlane, Bate, & Kyriakidou, 2004). Over the past decade more attention has been given to translation of knowledge to practice. The Canadian Institute of Health defines knowledge translation as "the synthesis, exchange and application of knowledge by relevant stakeholders to accelerate the benefits of global and local innovation in strengthening health systems and improving people's health" (CIHR, 2005, para 2).

Critics such as Harrison have argued that the evidence-based movement, "... centres on the assumption that valid and reliable knowledge is mainly to be obtained through the accumulation of research conducted by experts according to strict scientific criteria...and the distillation of such findings into protocols and guidelines" (Harrison, 2002, p. 469). It is argued that the evidence-based medicine movement in health care, and the increasing use of guidelines, has led to an increase in 'proceduralisation', with a greater number of 'tick lists' and compliance procedures and quality approaches such as audit and review to ensure the implementation of evidence-based procedures (Attree, 2005). Attree (2005) argues that the impact of the 'scientific-bureaucratic' or top-down approach to managing change in practice settings has met with dissatisfaction amongst staff with little uptake of evidence. More recently, Greenhalgh and Sietsewieringa

(2011) noted that little has changed and they are critical of what they see as traditional evidence translation models and argue for a broader approach such as that "found in the non-medical disciplines such as sociology and organization science where knowledge is conceptualized as being (for example) 'created', 'constructed', 'embodied', 'performed' and 'collectively negotiated' – and also as being value-laden and tending to serve the vested interests of dominant élites" (p. 502). These authors propose that applying a wider range of ideas and concepts would allow us to research the link between knowledge and practice in a more critical way.

We propose that ethnographic methods, particularly observations of practice, are a useful approach to achieve this understanding. Ethnographers focus on observing actions and interactions, linguistic and cultural manifestations such as signs, symbols, rules and rituals, relationships and conflicts or contradictions that may cast light on a specific social situation or problem (Emerson, 2009). Importantly, the ethnographer also examines and synthesises the perspectives of both the observer and the observed (Hammersley and Atkinson, 2007).

In our ethnographic projects we have used a critical lens to interpret midwifery and CFH nursing practice, and have found that frameworks and concepts from Michel Foucault, a French theorist and historian, are useful to explain practice. These concepts, including knowledge, disciplinary power, surveillance and resistance, can help to expose the individual and institutional practices that may influence the uptake of evidence into practice and to foster the development of a positive relationship between women/families and health professionals.

Approach and methods including summary of our studies

Between the years 2008 and 2013 we conducted or supervised five ethnographic projects, three of which are completed and published. Two of these studies were funded by the Australian Research Council Linkage programme. These studies all focused on exploring and understanding midwifery and or CFH nursing practice and the findings told us a lot about the nature and context of current maternity services in Australia and the impact of organisational culture on the individual practices of midwives and CFH nurses. A description of the three studies that we examine in this chapter is presented in Table 5.1 (pp. 78-81).

In this chapter we have undertaken an interpretive synthesis of our published findings. Interpretive synthesis is described by Campbell et al. (2011, p. 8) as an "approach to the synthesis of qualitative research, and has as its specific aim the achievement of the developmental goal of qualitative synthesis in terms of producing interpretations that go beyond individual studies and thus contribute to conceptual and theoretical development in the field". The output is, therefore, a new interpretation or theory that goes beyond the findings of any individual study. While some of the techniques we used are informed by meta-ethnography (Noblit & Hare, 1988), we have not strictly conducted a meta-ethnographic synthesis.

In preparing this chapter we first reviewed our published papers, extracting the key themes and data samples. We then proceeded to group these themes using headings such as 'approach to practice' (directive, the expert or technocrat, task-focused, woman-centred, flexible); 'under surveillance' (woman or professional); 'environment' (design of facility, policy directives). In the final stage of synthesis, we applied key concepts from the work of Foucault (knowledge, disciplinary power, regulation and monitoring, surveillance and resistance) to reorganise the data to 'tell a story' about the power of the Institution in shaping midwifery and CFH nursing practice and the opportunities that skilled midwives and CFH nurses found to work in woman-centred and flexible ways within the current maternity system in Australia.

Did we observe evidence in practice?

It is important to consider briefly the evidence base for the three practices we studied and to report on the degree to which we observed evidence-based practice. The first study detailed in Table 5.1 examined the process and impact of routine psychosocial assessment and depression screening. In NSW and increasingly in other Australian States and Territories and internationally, health services are implementing routine screening for risk factors associated with poor mental health in pregnancy and after birth (beyondblue: the national depression initiative, 2011; NSW Health, 2009), including screening for domestic violence. Further information about the evidence for routine psychosocial assessment is provided in Box 5.1. Our aim was to observe midwives and nurses to examine if and how routine screening was implemented. Rollans et al. (2013c) reported that all midwives observed in the 34 antenatal booking visits delivered the psychosocial assessment questions, including depression screening and screening

---

BOX 5.1 A brief overview of the evidence base for the midwifery and CFH nursing practices included in this chapter

STUDY 1: ROUTINE PSYCHOSOCIAL ASSESSMENT AND DEPRESSION SCREENING

Mental health problems in the perinatal period (pregnancy to first postnatal year) are a major public health issue with significant morbidity and costs for mother, infant, and family. To identify women at risk and offer appropriate services, universal psychosocial assessment during pregnancy is recommended as 'best practice' by the National Health and Medical Research Council (NHMRC-endorsed national guidelines) (beyondblue: the national depression initiative, 2011) and mandated in NSW health policy (NSW Health, 2009).

STUDY 2: PHYSIOLOGICAL BIRTH POSITIONS

Individual studies including randomised controlled trials and a meta-analysis report the physical and psychological benefits for women when they are able to adopt physiological positions in labour, and birth in an upright position of their choice. Women who utilise upright positions during labour have a shorter duration of the first (Lawrence et al., 2013) and second stage of labour (Gupta et al., 2012), experience less intervention, and report less severe pain and increased satisfaction with their childbirth experience than women in a semi-recumbent or supine/lithotomy position. Increased blood loss during third stage is the only disadvantage identified but this may be due to increased perineal oedema associated with upright positions. In NSW State government policy 'Towards Normal Birth' indicates that physiological birth positions should be encouraged.

STUDY 3: SUPPORTING WOMEN TO BREASTFEED

The National Health and Medical Research Council of Australia (NHMRC) endorsed the WHO/UNICEF strategy recommending infants be exclusively breastfed for the first six months and continue to be breastfed following the introduction of solid foods until at least 12 months of age (National Health and Medical Research Council, 2003). In NSW the State policy 'Breastfeeding in NSW: Promotion, Protection and Support' (2011) endorses these recommendations and supports the implementation of initiatives outlined in the Australian National Breastfeeding Strategy 2010–2015 including the implementation of the BFHI. The Cochrane review on breastfeeding support provides level 1 evidence of the improvements in breastfeeding exclusivity and duration from both lay support, and a combination of professional and lay support (Renfrew et al., 2012). Two recent meta-syntheses of breastfeeding support clearly outline what women find to be positive or helpful in professional and peer support (Virginia Schmied, Sarah Beake, Athena Sheehan, Christine McCourt, & Fiona Dykes, 2011; McInnes & Chambers, 2008, p. 422), particularly that professionals who engage in an 'authentic' way, demonstrating empathy, listening, taking time, and sharing the experience with the woman, provide facilitative breastfeeding support. The most helpful supportive styles adopted by health professionals included observing a complete feed, and confidence building (McInnes & Chambers, 2008, p. 418).

TABLE 5.1 Overview of the three ethnographic studies

Study 1

The perinatal journey: the process and impact of psychosocial assessment.
Mellanie Rollans, Virginia Schmied, Lynn Kemp and Tanya Meade

Study aim

This study aimed to examine and understand the meanings midwives, CFHNs and women make of the process of psychosocial assessment and depression screening undertaken during pregnancy and following birth.

Objectives: Describe the approaches (actions and interactions) that midwives and CFHNs take to psychosocial assessment and depression screening.

Examine midwives' and CFHNs' experiences and perceptions of the assessment process.

Explore women's experiences of being asked the psychosocial assessment questions – and how this influences women's responses.

Identify how the dynamics of these interactions facilitate or hinder the assessment and screening process and the potential for women to engage in ongoing support services or interventions.

Setting and participants

Setting:

Two maternity units and related community health services in NSW, Australia.

Participants:

34 women recruited at their first antenatal booking visit (14 to 20 weeks pregnancy).

Health professionals: total 110

25 midwives

2 student midwives

83 child and family health nurses.

Data collection

Observations:

34 observations of psychosocial assessment and depression screening at the antenatal booking visit.

20 observations of psychosocial assessment at the first postnatal home visit by a CFHN or in the CFHN clinic.

54 brief interviews: immediately following observation with midwife or CFHN.

Interviews with 31 women 2 to 4 weeks after the antenatal booking visit either by phone or face-to face.

Interviews with 29 women after birth either face-to-face or by phone.

2 focus groups with 18 midwives and 4 focus groups with 83 CFHNs.

Data analysis

Content analysis:

Content analysis was applied to the data from the observational tool (4D&4R) which provided categories or domains for what was being observed during interactions.

Thematic analysis:

Involved multiple readings of the data followed by identification and labelling of concepts and development of preliminary themes. Emerging concepts and themes were constantly compared with others and refined. This process resulted in identification of major themes for each of the data sets, antenatal, postnatal and the women's data.

Key findings/themes

Midwives and CFHNs varied in the approach taken to psychosocial assessment; some adopted a flexible approach and others were more process driven relying on the structured tools. Health professionals emphasised relationship-based approach and the importance of developing rapport with the women to establish comfort prior to assessment. Midwives and CFHNs experienced tensions conducting assessment which may partly be explained by the varying interpretations of the NSW SFE policy recommendations. Overall, women perceived the assessment questions were important; however, some experienced discomfort, surprise and felt unprepared to be asked these questions. Women who disclosed previous negative life events, such as child sexual abuse, were distressed by this experience but appeared to comply with the assessment process.

Publications

Rollans, M., Schmied, V., Kemp, L., & Meade, T. (2012). 'We just ask some questions...': the process of antenatal psychosocial assessment by midwives. *Midwifery*, 29(8), 935–942.

Rollans, M., Schmied, V., Kemp, L., & Meade, T. (2012). Negotiating policy in practice: child and family health nurses approach to the process of postnatal psychosocial assessment. *BMC Health Services Research* 13(1).

Rollans, M., Schmied, V., Kemp, L., & Meade, T. (2012). 'Digging over that old ground': an Australian perspective of women's experience of psychosocial assessment and depression screening in pregnancy and following birth. *BMC Women's Health* 13(1).

Study 2

Facilitating physiological birth positioning in three different birth settings: An exploration into facilitators and inhibitors

Hannah Dahlen, Virginia Schmied, Soo Downe and Sally Tracy

Study aim

To explore how physiological birth positioning is facilitated by midwives and experienced by women in three main settings in NSW, Australia (home, birth centre and delivery ward).

Setting and participants

Setting

Delivery wards and birth centres in two maternity units in NSW, Australia as well as the homes of 6 women participants.

Participants

Total 118 participants: 25 women who were at low risk for birth complications, 11 homebirth midwives, 10 midwives working in birth centres, 16 midwives working in delivery wards, 21 midwifery consultants, 25 student midwives and 10 newly graduated midwives.

Data collection

Observations of 25 women during labour and birth: 6 at home; 10 in the 2 birth centres; 9 in the two delivery wards).

Interviews with 25 women. Focus groups (1 group with 11 homebirth midwives; 2 groups with 10 birth centre midwives; 2 groups with 16 delivery ward midwives; 1 with midwifery consultants; 2 with student midwives). Large group discussions with midwives in 2 workshops, one in the UK and one in Australia.

Table 5.1 continued

Data analysis
Thematic analysis (as above)

Key findings/themes
When women give birth they run a gauntlet. The more women interact with the mainstream maternity system the more they come into contact with the gauntlet. The gauntlet has the least influence in the home and most influence in the hospital delivery ward. Physiological birth positions (PBP) are either facilitated or inhibited as the result of complex interconnections and interactions between the environment (which can buffer women from the gauntlet) and the philosophical framework of women and midwives (which can facilitate or inhibit PBP). It is this dynamic interconnection that determines whether women and midwives will survive or become the gauntlet and whether PBP will be experienced. PBP is strongly linked to normal birth.

Publications
Priddis, H., Dahlen, H., & Schmied, V. (2011). Juggling instinct and fear: an ethnographic study of facilitators and inhibitors of physiological birth positioning in two different birth settings. *International Journal of Childbirth,* 1(4), 227–241.
Dahlen, H., Schmied, V., Downe, S., Tracy, S., Dowling, H., Upton, A., et al. (2010). Facilitating physiological birth positioning in three different birth settings: an exploration into facilitators and inhibitors. PSANZ. *Journal of Paediatrics and Child Health*, 46 (Suppl.1), 57–96.
Priddis, H., Dahlen, H., & Schmied, V. (2012). What are the facilitators, inhibitors, and implications of birth positioning? A review of the literature. *Women and Birth*, 25(2), 100–106.

Study 3
Mining for liquid gold: An analysis of the language and practices of midwives when interacting with women who are establishing breastfeeding.
Elaine Burns, Virginia Schmied, Jennifer Fenwick and Athena Sheehan

Study aim
To study the nature, and impact, of midwifery language and practices during early breastfeeding support.
Objectives
Describe and analyse the language and practices employed by midwives when supporting breastfeeding women during the first week after birth.
Identify the patterns and components of verbal and non-verbal interactions which facilitate or inhibit support for breastfeeding women.
Analyse the impact of these interactions on women in the post-birth period.

Setting and participants
Setting
Two maternity units in NSW, Australia.
Participants
36 midwives participated in the observation of practice, and a further 11 midwives participated in an individual interview whilst 35 participated in a focus group interview.
77 women participated in the observational component of the study in the first week after birth (45 having had their first baby; 32 subsequent baby).

Data collection

85 observations of interactions between midwives and women (total 33 hours of recorded interaction – 65 interactions occurred in hospital postnatal unit and 20 interactions in the woman's home).

23 interviews were conducted at 4 to 6 weeks after birth with women who participated in the interactions (21 in the woman's home; 1 by phone and 1 in the postnatal unit at the woman's request).

11 interviews with senior staff (managers, midwifery educators, senior lactation consultants and senior clinicians).

4 focus groups with 35 midwives and lactation consultants (2 focus groups in each maternity unit).

Data analysis

Poststructuralist approach and critical discourse analysis – a three-dimensional approach incorporating the interplay between text, discourse practices and context.

Key findings/themes

Analysis revealed three discourses in the language and practices of midwives. In the dominant discourse, 'Mining for Liquid Gold', midwives held great reverence for breastmilk as 'liquid gold' and prioritised breastfeeding as the mechanism for transferring breastmilk.

In the second discourse, 'not rocket science', breastfeeding was constructed as 'natural' or 'easy' – something that all women could do if they were committed. In this approach, midwives tended to leave women to 'their own devices' unless they requested help.

The third discourse constructed 'breastfeeding as a relationship' between mother and infant. In this minority discourse, women were viewed as knowledgeable about their needs and those of their infant. Midwives facilitated communication and built confidence.

Publications

Burns, E., Fenwick, J., Sheehan, A., & Schmied, V. (2013). Mining for liquid gold: midwifery language and practices associated with early breastfeeding support. *Maternal and Child Nutrition*, 9(1), 57–73.

Burns, E., Schmied, V., Fenwick, J., & Sheehan, A. (2012). Liquid gold from the milk bar: constructions of breastmilk and breastfeeding women in the language and practices of midwives. *Social Science and Medicine*, 75(10), 1737–1745.

Fenwick, J., Burns, E., Sheehan, A., & Schmied, V. (2012). 'We only talk about breastfeeding': a discourse analysis of infant feeding messages in antenatal group-based education. *Midwifery*, published online S0266–6138(12)00038 for domestic violence. This was expected as the computer database used to record women's information had mandatory fields. In 29 out of the 34 booking visits the midwife provided an introduction to the psychosocial questions at least once during the interview, either at the beginning of the assessment or prior to asking the questions. In 21 interactions a rationale for asking the questions was provided and in two-thirds the privacy act was read as required prior to asking the domestic violence questions. In all (20 out of 20) of the observed interactions following birth, the CFH nurse used the Edinburgh Postnatal Depression Scale (EPDS) to screen for possible depression. In contrast, only one nurse at site 1 undertook the structured psychosocial assessment as recommended by the State policy, while at the second site, the assessment was completed in 9 of the 10 observed interactions. At site 1, screening for domestic violence was conducted on four occasions and at site 2, all the CFHNs undertook domestic violence screening as outlined in the policy (Rollans et al., 2013b).

Our second study examined the facilitators and inhibitors of physiological birth positioning (see Table 5.1). Level 1 evidence supports the benefits of upright positions during first and second stage of labour (Gupta, Hofmeyr, & Shehmar, 2012). In our study, all women who gave birth at home were upright and off the bed (100 per cent). Five out of six gave birth in water. Seven out of ten women in the birth centres also gave birth upright and one woman gave birth semi-recumbent in water, with four giving birth on a bed. In the delivery wards two out of nine women gave birth in an upright forwards leaning position and nine gave birth on a bed (Dahlen et al., 2010; Priddis, Dahlen, & Schmied, 2011). The amount of time women spent semi-recumbent or recumbent in labour was examined. We found no women at home spent any time in this position. Women in Birth Centre 1 spent 3.4 per cent and in Birth Centre 2 18.7 per cent of time in a semi-recumbent position. In Delivery Ward 1, 32 per cent of time and in Delivery Ward 2, 75.53 per cent of time was spent semi-recumbent. We also observed no vaginal examinations at home and 18 vaginal examinations for the 10 women in the birth centre and 21 vaginal examinations for the 9 women in the delivery ward (Dahlen et al., 2010).

The third study focused on the language and practices of midwives in interactions with women around breastfeeding in the first week after birth (see Table 5.1). Internationally, there is a high level of policy support for breastfeeding and there is level 1 evidence that support from lay supporters and professionals results in higher initiation and duration of breastfeeding (Renfrew, McCormick, Wade, Quinn, & Dowswell, 2012). However, two meta-syntheses demonstrate that it is 'how' that support is provided that makes the difference (McInnes & Chambers, 2008; Schmied, Beake, Sheehan, McCourt, & Dykes, 2011). Burns et al. (2013) reported that midwives assumed one of three approaches when they supported women with breastfeeding. In the first and dominant approach in 68 out of 85 (80 per cent) of the interactions, midwives demonstrated a high level of support for breastfeeding but this support had a technocratic focus, ensuring that babies got breastmilk by whatever means were necessary, often with disruption to the mother–infant relationship. A smaller group of midwives in 9 out of 85 interactions (11 per cent), did not value breastfeeding support in the same way, and tended to leave the woman to her own devices. In the third discourse, breastfeeding was approached as a relationship between the woman and her baby and was observed in 8 out of 85 (9 per cent) of the interactions. Here the language and practices of midwives genuinely facilitated communication and built the breastfeeding woman's confidence (see Table 5.1).

Knowledge and disciplinary power: the midwife and nurse as expert

At the basis of Foucault's work is an understanding that power operates at "a micro, local, and covert level, through sets of specific practices" (Peterson & Bunton, 1997, p. xi) and is not limited to overt instances of oppression from authoritative agencies such as governments, Foucault used the term 'biopower' to describe the way "power relations work in and through the body" (Lupton, 1995, p. 6). Biopower acts on two dimensions. First, constituting the individual body particularly through individual interactions with health professionals (Fahy & Parratt, 2006; Lupton, 1995). Second, biopower acts as a *disciplinary power* that regulates the population, for example through the control of fertility, management of health and illness and corporeal habits and customs, particularly the control of sexuality. Disciplinary power is fundamentally about manipulating and training bodies, and regulating behaviour. It works by establishing norms which people try to live up to. Whilst these disciplinary norms may be seen as originating from institutions, schools, factories, hospitals, prisons, they are usually so well integrated into the fabric of society that people experience them as natural or innate.

A number of authors have applied concepts from Foucault to understand how authoritative knowledge and disciplinary power manifest within health care institutions and their services, such as maternity and CFH nursing services, and they have examined the role of the health professional as an agent of the state (Appleton & Cowley, 2008; Fahy & Parratt, 2006; Marcellus, 2005; Peckover, 2003; Scamell, 2011; Wilson, 2001). Health professionals in maternity and CFH services engage in 'routine health surveillance' of the particular population in their care. Even routine health surveillance can be viewed as 'watchful waiting', and of exercising 'power over' others, resulting in subtle coercion to achieve alignment with authoritative knowledge (Marcellus, 2005). A more focused gaze on the woman such as in psychosocial assessment and depression screening, to detect signs of psychological and social problems or the potential for child abuse or neglect, can lead to the uncomfortable alignment of midwives and nurses as the 'health police' (Crisp & Lister, 2004; Marcellus, 2005; Peckover, 2003). As a result, a tension can develop between the health professional providing a supportive service to vulnerable women and families and in fact exercising a 'policing' role, where the home environment and parenting practices are observed through a "disciplinary lens" (Roche et al., 2005). Indeed our work examining the language and practices of midwives supporting women who are breastfeeding was initiated because of a widespread discourse depicting midwives as the 'breast police' or as 'nipple Nazis'. The study findings revealed that an overzealous approach to monitoring and surveying women's competency with breastfeeding resulted in negative experiences of breastfeeding support and in turning some women away from breastfeeding (Burns et al., 2012).

Disciplinary power in midwifery and CFH nursing practice

In focus groups and interviews, midwives and CFH nurses emphasised the importance of building relationships and working in partnership with the women and families that they supported in pregnancy, birth, the postnatal and early childhood period. Yet our observations of practice often revealed a different story. Across the three studies midwives and CFH nurses positioned themselves in different ways, depending upon the individual philosophy of practice or to use a Foucauldian term, they drew on different discourses. A small number of midwives were observed to be practising within a woman-centred philosophy, demonstrating the capacity to be flexible in their approach as they responded to women's individual needs. The majority, however, established and maintained their position as the 'expert', showing greater allegiance to the needs of the institution and the broader health system than they did to the individual women and families in their care. In this approach midwives or nurses appeared to hold power, often taking a directive approach, cajoling the woman to comply, 'doing for' or taking over. Women thus assumed a 'docile' role, acquiescing to the wish or demand of the professional. We also found some professionals fluctuated in their approach, at times being 'with woman' and/or family-centred and other times taking on the expert role. For example, in the birth positions study we found that midwives (and women) assumed one of three positions: a physiological (evidence-based) philosophy of birth positioning, a 'going with the flow' which depended on the woman's preferences or the environment they worked/birthed in or a directive, 'technocratic approach' (Dahlen et al., 2010). These positions aligned directly with the findings from the establishing breastfeeding study where the three distinct positions included a technocratic expert positioning, a 'not rocket science' or going-with-the-flow positioning and a relationship-focused position which prioritised the mother–baby relationship and the midwife–woman relationship (Burns et al., 2013). We noted in these studies that the different approaches were present across all settings – hospital, home and community – although private or caseload midwives supporting women at home invariably were more woman-centred and physiological in their approach.

Midwife and nurse as the expert

In the postnatal unit, Burns et al. reported that the technocratic 'expert' midwives were "inclined to provide long spiels of information about breastfeeding to women" (Burns et al., 2012, p. 1742), in order to fill an assumed knowledge deficit. It appeared that the more 'knowledgeable' the midwife was, the more information they wanted to pass on to the woman. This was often regardless of whether the woman had indicated a need for the information (Burns et al., 2013). In addition to giving information, supervision by the expert was considered necessary to ensure that the baby was 'getting on right' and was not causing 'damage' to the breasts. Midwives often appeared to be the teacher providing information in a directive manner to the 'novice' breastfeeding woman. In addition, the language used by midwives often gave the impression that women were being 'tested' to 'check' if they had learned the necessary skills (Burns et al., 2012).

We observed that midwives or nurses who adopt the role as 'expert' were inclined to be directive, issuing instructions to women. For example, in the illustration below from Rollans et al., the woman was instructed to complete tasks such as filling in the EPDS:

> M2: (hands the woman the EPDS) I want you to do this.
> W8: Do you want me to tick?
> M2: (explains hastily) Underline, underline.
>
> (Rollans et al., 2013c, p. 939)

When observed in breastfeeding interactions, some midwives dominated the interactions and 'took over' from women, physically accessing and touching the breast, often without seeking the woman's consent. We observed that some midwives commenced breastfeeding interactions with women 'ready for action' with gloves in hand poised to provide non-evidence-based 'hands-on' assistance with breastfeeding support (Burns et al., 2013). No time was spent ascertaining the needs of the woman or infant. Using a 'hands on' (midwife attaching the baby for the woman) approach to 'show' how to 'best' attach an infant led to midwives taking control over the woman's body and resulted in women assuming a passive and docile position:

> Midwife: Let me get some gloves. We'll see if we can get the baby on …
> [then later]
> Midwife: I'm a little bit quicker … (at putting the baby on)
> Midwife: You sit there and I'll do it.
> (The midwife placed her gloved hands onto the woman and attached the baby to the woman's breast. The woman was non-verbally instructed to keep her hands out of the way.)
>
> (Interaction 72) (Burns et al., 2013, p. 61)

Burns et al. reported that the expert midwife believed they 'had the knack' to get the baby on the breast, "Midwife: Probably at this stage we'll just get it out and get it into her, because there is a bit of a knack to it and if you were up it's easier you know if you were standing in front of a mirror you can sort of see where to squeeze ..." (Burns et al., 2013, p. 62). Having the 'knack' was a prized skill that afforded some midwives a sense of status within their professional peer group. The following field note was recorded after a midwife returned from helping another midwife attach a difficult infant: "... just got 12 on the breast, fussy little bugger, naughty boy, got him on though ..." (Burns et al., 2013, p. 62). 'Doing for' the woman rather than sharing with the woman the skills and knowledge to enable her to undertake this activity herself was common, and was often used as a device to save time.

In a similar way, midwives working in the delivery ward environment reported that they 'invade' the woman's space:

> Yeah, you're doing stuff. You're doing stuff. Constantly in her ear, I'm just going do this, I'm just going to do that. And it's virtually every ten minutes at least you're going, I'm just going to do this. Can you just move back a little because I've just got to put this in here? It's constant interruption. (DW Midwife)
>
> (Dahlen et al., 2010)

In the physiological birth positioning study and the breastfeeding interactions study, midwives had a set of 'tools' (Burns et al., 2013) or 'bag of tricks' (Priddis et al., 2011) which were used as rhetorical devices or strategies to meet the midwife's goals for evidence-based practice. For example, some midwives used these strategies to persuade individual women to go along with their plans. Midwives reported that they consciously cajoled women into assuming physiological birth positions. For example,

> Putting the idea into the lady's head as if it's her decision. So she thinks she's empowered, really you've fed her the information that she needs, but she's made the decision on her own to, okay. How about I try this then? You feed her all the information and then she makes her own choice. (DW Midwife)
>
> (Priddis et al., 2011, p. 234)

Regulation, monitoring and control policies, procedures and ticking the box

Foucault has shown us how our culture attempts to normalise individuals through increasingly rationalised means, "turning them into meaningful subjects and docile objects" (Dreyfus & Rabinow, 1983, p. xxvii). In his work titled *Discipline and Punish* (Foucault, 1977) advances that the body has been approached as an object to be analysed and separated into its constituent parts. Through what Foucault calls disciplinary technology, found in the daily practices of institutions, he describes how the body as a target of power has been manipulated, shaped, and trained, forging a 'docile body' (Foucault, 1977, p.

136). Whether in school, factory or hospital, many people become caught within the regulations, voluntarily acquiescing to the timetabling and examinations through which discipline can be imposed (Foucault, 1977). Institutions, such as hospitals, have become large efficiency-driven machines that are increasingly controlled by procedures and routines (Smeets, Gribnau, & van der Ven, 2011). Proceduralisation leads to the multiplication of control systems, so that the solution to minimising errors is to improve and continually increase policies and procedures in order to stop problems from recurring. The constant and increasingly invasive monitoring of women during pregnancy is a powerful example of the manifestation of this disciplinary technology.

In the regulated and monitored environment of an acute hospital maternity unit, we found that many midwives were focused on obtaining, recording and reporting on the 'tasks' required of them and demonstrated little flexibility to address the individual needs of women. In the first antenatal encounter, some midwives intent on completing the task, ignored key elements of relationship building, such as introductions (Davis & Day, 2010). Rollans observed that some midwives or nurses moved immediately to the 'business' addressing administrative tasks such as previous blood tests or obtaining contact details (Rollans et al., 2013c). These midwives took a very 'matter of fact' approach to psychosocial assessment, indicating to women that this was a job that had to be done, "we ask all women these questions" (Rollans et al., 2013c), "there is a lot of paperwork" (Rollans et al., 2013b) and stating in focus groups that it was just about getting the job done. We also noted that these midwives focused on the computer during the encounter, only sometimes or rarely maintaining eye contact with the woman.

If a woman resisted requests for psychosocial information, some midwives would press on regardless. For example, one woman when asked about previous abuse as a child requested the midwife refer to her medical records where she had previously disclosed childhood trauma:

> M3: So as a child were you hurt or abused in any way either physically, sexually or emotionally?
> W4: Yes.
> M3: Did you want to tell me about that?
> W4: Isn't it in my file from last time?
> M3: No… Well I haven't read it… you can tell me about it now?
>
> (Rollans et al., 2013a, p. 10)

In the field notes the researcher noted that "the woman described her experience reluctantly" (Rollans et al., 2013a).

In the breastfeeding interactions we observed, one group of midwives prioritised other tasks such as routine observations over support with breastfeeding. Some midwives believed that breastfeeding was 'not rocket science' and that if a woman needed help she would ask. One midwife described organising her work for the shift in the following way:

> ...first I'd have a diagnosis, then I'd check the notes and see if there's anything else that I need to know. Then I'd prioritise who needs medications, who needs them when, who is the most dependent, which would be surgical patients, which would be a Caesar. Who needs to get up..., who needs my help the most, physical help, and who needs that nursing care type thing first. There's no way you can do it any other way, because if you try to go well let's just do the breastfeeding first, we'd have patients sitting in the bed all day. So I'd probably go and do the nursing things first, knowing that there's midwifery things to do and then I'd work my way through the midwifery things.... (SSIV3)
>
> (Burns et al., 2013, p. 66)

In this extract, the midwife is clearly privileging the 'nursing' tasks such as medications and routine observations that must be documented (and potentially audited) over midwifery care related to breastfeeding. In addition, technocratic 'expert midwives' tended to approach breastfeeding interactions as being about the 'breast' and 'nutrition' and not about the woman. The focus was on 'this particular' breastfeed and 'this particular' baby and interactions with the woman lacked any form of 'checking in' with her about previous breastfeeding experiences or previous solutions to breastfeeding difficulties.

Taking this further, we reported in our birth positions study that the institution acted as 'a gauntlet' that both women and midwives had to navigate in order to achieve a normal birth. By this we mean that a range of non-evidence-based institutional policies and procedures (e.g. routine admission cardiotocograph (CTG), four-hourly vaginal examinations) combined with the individual philosophical framework of midwives (and women), limited midwives' capacity to support women to use physiological birth positions and to achieve a normal birth. We have described the 'gauntlet' as having the least influence in the home and most influence in the institution – the hospital delivery ward (Dahlen et al., 2010; Priddis et al., 2011). However, the birth centre provided an intermediate space in which the complex dynamics of acceptance of, or resistance to the gauntlet, were most evident among women and midwives, with varying consequences for physiological birth positioning, and for other labour outcomes. Midwives noted in the focus group discussion that particularly in a delivery ward where 'the gauntlet' was most intense it was difficult to see birth as a normal event, when intervention in birth was high and normal birth less common.

> I think we lose touch with the normal. We lose touch with what's normal in what is a normal physiological event for most women but in a unit like this it is very easy to go down the path of thinking it is not normal and I think that is how the doctors think, they don't deal with enough normal. (DW midwives focus group)
>
> (Dahlen et al., 2010)

Doing the right thing: self-surveillance by midwives and nurses

Above we have described how midwives and nurses use their knowledge and disciplinary power to direct and monitor the behaviour of women in order to ensure compliance with the institutional procedures and/or the preferences of individual practitioners. This use of 'expertise' or authoritative knowledge has been well described by researchers investigating contemporary maternity care (Davis Floyd, 1997; Jordan, 1992; Katz Rothman, 1989). However, we also observed that midwives monitored their own behaviour and actions as they feared reprimand from others. Midwives in all three studies were concerned that their practices were being observed or monitored by others and as a consequence midwives then participated in self-monitoring their own behaviour.

According to Foucault, *disciplinary power* which emanates from superior knowledge claims, can produce a submissive subject position, whereby the individual becomes complicit in their own surveillance and control (Sarup, 1989). Individuals become 'self-governing' subjects who monitor and control their own behaviour to 'fit' within the social constraints (Foucault, 1977). This was particularly well illustrated in Foucault's work on prisons and the notion of the Panopticon (Foucault, 1977). Foucault describes that in the prison one of the main disciplinary techniques employed was surveillance. The development of a panopticon, a circular building, allowed viewing of prisoners' cells from all areas in the prison. Prisoners could never be certain where or when they were being watched. Therefore those who were jailed had to monitor and regulate their own behaviour according to the rules of the prison. This form of self-governing in prisons paralleled the form of control expected of individuals within society.

In the birth positions study, midwives working in both the birth centre and delivery suite indicated that they were required to adjust or adapt their philosophy of care to comply with the system. Midwives described protecting themselves from the system and ramifications when birth deviated from normal.

> Midwives are protecting themselves from the gauntlet they would need to run through if someone did "fall off the perch". (BC Midwife)
>
> (Priddis et al., 2011, p. 235)

While midwives in the birth centre did not undertake frequent clinical assessments of the women in labour, they nonetheless felt under surveillance and experienced pressure to conduct routine observations:

> We are constantly under scrutiny—like they are waiting for us to fail. (BC Midwife)
>
> (Priddis et al., 2011, p. 235)

> Sometimes you think they're going to come to me and say, "Why didn't you VE her at that time and not"—it's a bit scary, that they're going to come to you and point things, "why didn't you do it"? (BC Midwife)
>
> (Priddis et al., 2011, p. 235)

We observed, on a number of occasions in these studies, that midwives and nurses sometimes appeared to act against women's wishes in order to protect themselves from criticism from colleagues, management or the medical profession. Rollans et al. observed instances when a woman, after disclosing an emotional or social issue, stated that that she did not want or require a referral to other another service such as social work, yet the midwife or CFH nurse insisted that the referral was necessary and proceeded with the protocol, informing the woman that she could refuse the service when the social worker or other staff member contacted them (Rollans et al., 2013a). This practice implied that the midwife or nurse was concerned that if she had not referred the women, then down the track she may be blamed for not complying with the protocol.

Environment shapes practice

We observed that the environment itself played a powerful role in shaping the actions of midwives, nurses and women. In each of these studies the environment, both the architectural design and furnishings/equipment, influenced how care was provided and how the woman experienced care. Stark contrasts were observed between care provided in the institution (antenatal clinic, delivery suite, postnatal ward) and care in the home, community clinic or birth centre. In particular, care provided in the institution was governed by the rules of the institution and was owned by the staff.

The design or layout of the birthing facilities was crucial. For example, in one study site the birth centre was located next to the delivery suite and to enter the birth centre women had to walk past the admission room. Because of this proximity, women were likely to be required to enter the admission room and to have an admission CTG, which is a non-evidence-based intervention. Dahlen et al. reported that 9 out of 10 women booked into the birth centre and observed for the study had an admission CTG (Priddis et al., 2011).

We observed that the birth centre environment was much more conducive to or facilitative of upright and forward-leaning birth positions because of ease of access to equipment such as a birthing stool, bean bags, and mats on the floor, and an absence of continuous electronic fetal monitoring equipment. One woman in the study stated "I think, anyway, I'd tried everything in the room, so that was the last thing (birth stool) ..." (BC Woman) (Priddis et al., 2011, p. 234). In contrast the delivery suite environment was clinical in appearance; the bed was the central feature of the room, implying that the woman would use the bed for most of her stay there.

There might just be a bed in the middle of the room, and nothing else, and then they can't get up and move around as much as they want, if they wanted a bean bag or something like that, because it might be hidden in the corner or it might have half beans full in it… or there is no bath in the room… some rooms at our hospital don't even have a bath in them so that is just not an option if we're full. (new graduate midwife)

(Priddis et al., 2011 p 235).

The most positive experiences were reported by women who birthed at home. Here women were in their own environment and clearly in charge there. There was far less talking in the homebirth environment than in hospital and the focus appeared to be completely on the woman, with midwives guided by the women rather than directing the process (Dahlen et al., 2010). Midwives in the homebirth and birth centre environment saw their role more as 'holding the space' for women to have a normal birth. This was reinforced by the lack of medical equipment, the homelike environment and shared physiological paradigm. Women were aware of the midwives' low-key presence.

I guess she just stood outside and realised when I was doing my deep breathing as to how frequently the contractions were coming. She didn't interfere. The lights were off. Everything was perfect…I would only realise that she'd been in the room when I'd realise that the CD would then start again. (BC Woman)

(Dahlen et al., 2010)

Fahy and Parratt drew on Foucault's work to theorise the birth room environment, describing a theory or 'Birth Territory'. In this theory, the midwife has a responsibility to 'guard' the birth territory for women – to ensure the environment is conducive to facilitating normal physiological birth. They identified two types of 'terrain', one a 'Sanctum' defined as "a homely environment designed to optimise the privacy, ease and comfort of the women; with access to facilities such as a bath" (Fahy & Parratt, 2006, p. 46), which protects the woman. The other is a 'surveillance room', "a clinical environment designed to facilitate surveillance of the woman and to optimise the ease and comfort of the staff" (Fahy & Parratt, 2006, p. 46). In the 'surveillance room' equipment that may be needed is on display and the bed dominates.

Resistance: building relationships to deliver evidence-based, woman-centred care

So far we have applied a range of Foucault's concepts to expose the powerful and often negative or repressive influence of disciplinary practices on the actions and interactions of midwives and nurses. Yet Foucault believes that if power was only repressive it would not survive, and nobody would accept it. Thus, while a discourse may offer a preferred form of subjectivity, a way of being and acting for example, as a midwife or CFH nurse, it also offers the possibility of reversal. A reversal of discourse enables the subject of that discourse to speak out in their own right, to position themselves in ulterior ways. Foucault asserts that "where there is power there is always resistance, one is always inside power, there is no escaping it" (Foucault, 1977, p. 94). In our studies, some midwives, nurses and women resisted the dominant discourses to facilitate the implementation of evidence-based practice for example, to facilitate physiological birth positions or alternatively to reject the 'proceduralist' or 'standardised governing of practice' by paying attention to the individual needs of the woman or families.

Woman-centred care, family-centred care and partnership are core principles of midwifery and CFH nursing practice. In midwifery texts, these concepts form the basis on which a midwife or CFH nurse (Hopwood, Fowler, Lee, Rossiter, & Bigsby, 2013) is able to deliver evidence-based interventions or healthcare and to support a woman to have a normal birth, to transition to motherhood, to establish breastfeeding and to care for her baby. This philosophy or discourse places women and their babies at the heart of midwifery practice (Renfrew et al., 2014) and the midwife–woman relationship is characterised by trust and respect (ten Hoope-Bender et al., 2014) and is exemplified in the following quote.

> You're working with them, they're trusting you and they're trusting themselves to be in the position that's most comfortable for them… trusting the mother means you also trust her to be in control and make decisions that are right for her. (Private midwife)
>
> (Dahlen et al., 2010).

Building relationships: taking time

Midwives who were woman-centred were observed spending time with women. They took time for introductions, interacting with the woman and her partner (if present) in an engaging way, often starting with general questions such as, 'How have things been going?'

> It's so important you know getting that first bit right. They're checking you out seeing if you're good enough and if they can trust you. So it's really important how you introduce yourself and what needs to be done.
>
> (Rollans et al., 2013b, p. 7)

In field notes Rollans et al. reported that a sense of friendliness and warmth was evidenced by soft facial gestures, soft or neutral tone of voice, smiling and a balance of eye contact between the computer and woman (Rollans et al., 2013b). These midwives and nurses took time to assess the situation and ask questions about the woman's thoughts and experience. When this occurred it appeared to facilitate a more collaborative approach to decision making and problem solving (Rollans et al., 2013b). Burns et al. reported that midwives who prioritised building a relationship with women "tended to begin their interactions with women by engaging in friendly 'chat' before enquiring about the areas the woman would like to discuss" (Burns et al., 2013, p. 67). They referred to midwives 'checking in' with women. This approach included enquiries about other aspects of her life and did not focus exclusively on breastfeeding. Women participants described this as a desire 'to know [their] story':

> She was great (the midwife). I would love to have bottled her and kept her but I had her in my life for two hours… . She wanted to know the story. She asked the story. So how did the birth go? She was the first person who asked who really listened to that story. (Int 12)
>
> (Burns et al., 2013, p. 67)

Valuing women and sharing power

When midwives adopted a woman-centred approach they communicated to the woman using verbal and non-verbal language that they had confidence in her ability to birth and to care for her infant, particularly to breastfeed. Some midwives sought the woman's own knowledge about her newborn infant, and these midwives used open-ended questions to gather woman-led information, for example, "What do you feel about your supply?" (Burns et al., 2013, p. 67). The support needed by the woman was gauged during a period of 'tuning in' to the woman's feelings and incorporated 'hands-off' breastfeeding support. However, if the woman indicated a desire for 'hands-on' assistance, or a demonstration from the midwife, this was also accommodated.

At times midwives and CFH nurses shared aspects of their own experience or perhaps simply how their day was going. On four occasions, Rollans et al. also observed that when a woman disclosed a personal story the midwife responded to the woman and then also reflected on her own experience and shared this with the women: "I know when that happened to me I was like totally not expecting it…" (Rollans et al., 2013c, p. 939). One CFHN in a clinic environment started the interaction in the following way: "Hi, how are you going?", the woman responded by asking the CFH nurse how she is; who then shared her story of the difficulties experienced getting to work that morning "I've had one of those mornings" (Rollans et al., 2013b, p. 7). In field notes it was documented that this appeared to put the family at ease as they laughed and enjoyed the CFH nurse's lightheartedness.

Manipulating the system to meet women's needs

We have described above the set of tools or bag of tricks that midwives employed to cajole or coerce women into complying with institution norms or practices. However, midwives also used their tools or tricks to manipulate the system to ensure women received evidence-based practice. In the birth positions study for example, midwives used their 'tricks' or strategies to facilitate physiological birth positioning. One midwife described:

> I've done an induction in delivery suite, and I made her stand up. Even with the CTG strapped on her belly, I got her up, and she delivered standing. (BC Midwife)

(Priddis et al., 2011, p. 234)

Similarly when undertaking psychosocial assessment, some midwives varied the wording or the order or the timing of the psychosocial questions from the structured computer-based questions. This appeared to assist the woman in understanding the questions, particularly if she was from a non-English-speaking background (Rollans et al., 2013c).

Conclusion

In this chapter we have synthesised the key findings from three ethnographic studies that examined specific midwifery and CFH nursing practices. Observations of care have been used for some time as a key element in professional development and leadership through a facilitated, action learning programme (Harrison, 2011; Harvey et al., 2002; Kitson, 2009). Yet arguably little has changed in either the context or mechanisms of care. In these studies, we used observations in a more critical way with a view to understanding local cultures and how players act and feel in this context and how power is distributed and exercised within the organisation.

We observed an innovation gap across the three practices in different settings, reflecting the inadequate integration of 'best-practice knowledge' into actual practice. By applying key concepts from the work of Foucault, we propose this innovation gap is linked to the way in which evidence-based practices are 'imposed' upon health practitioners (and consequently women and families) through a range of targets and performance measures. This was particularly so in the case of psychosocial assessment and depression screening and in provision of breastfeeding support. It was also clear that an alternative position existed, whereby evidence-based practice related to physiological birth positions was not supported in the acute care delivery ward environment in contrast to birth centres and in women's own homes.

Across all three studies, instead of evidence-based practice being, as Sackett describes, about the "compassionate use of individual patients' [in this case women's] predicaments, rights, and preferences in making clinical decisions about their care" (Sackett, 1997, p. 3), our synthesis indicates that the prime focus was on demonstrating that institutional requirements were met. We did report examples of resistance, where midwives and nurses demonstrated that they could be flexible or adapt their practice and environment to meet the needs of women and families. These health professionals prioritised the relationship they had with women and worked in partnership with women to implement evidence-based practice. As identified, shifting care from the institution to the community, particularly to the woman's home, changes the interactions and facilitates the development of a partnership.

Finally, this work demonstrates the futile nature of attempts to control evidence-based midwifery and CFH nursing practice from the top down by setting targets and performance indicators and increasing external control structures to drive through change. As Bilson and Thorpe explain "approaching the complex behaviour of human systems without properly understanding the theoretical basis for our actions, what might be called cybernetic wisdom, leads to frustration and in some cases harm" (Bilson & Thorpe, 2007, p. 937). Our analysis of our combined ethnographic work underscores the importance of taking a bottom-up and top-down approach to practice change and the value of respectful collaboration across professions, services and with consumers.

References

Appleton, J.V., & Cowley, S. (2008). Health visiting assessment processes under scrutiny: a case study of knowledge use during family health needs assessments. *International Journal of Nursing Studies, 45*(5), 682–696.

Attree, Moira. (2005). Nursing agency and governance: registered nurses perceptions. *Journal of Nursing Management, 13*(5), 387–396.

beyondblue: the national depression initiative. (2011). Clinical practice guidelines for depression and related disorders – anxiety, bipolar disorder and puerperal psychosis – in the perinatal period. Retrieved March 31st, 2011, from http://www.beyondblue.org.au/index.aspx?link_id=6.1246

Bilson, A., & Thorpe, D. (2007). Towards aesthetic seduction using emotional engagement and stories. *Kybernetes, 36*(7/8), 936–945.

Burns, E., Schmied, V., Fenwick, J., & Sheehan, A. (2012). Liquid gold from the milk bar: constructions of breastmilk and breastfeeding women in the language and practices of midwives. *Social Science and Medicine, 75*(10), 1737–1745.

Burns, E., Fenwick, J., Sheehan, A., & Schmied, V. (2013). Mining for liquid gold: midwifery language and practices associated with early breastfeeding support. *Maternal and Child Nutrition, 9*(1), 57–73.

Campbell, R., Pound, P., Morgan, M., Daker-White, G., Britten, N., Pill, R., … & Yardley, L. (2011) *Evaluating Meta Ethnography: Systematic Analysis and Synthesis of Qualitative Research.* Health Technology Assessment 15. London: NIHR Health Technology Assessment Programme.

CIHR, Canadian Institutes of Health Research. (2005). *About Knowledge Translation.* Ottawa: CIHR.

Crisp, Beth R., & Lister, Pam Green. (2004). Child protection and public health: nurses' responsibilities. *Journal of Advanced Nursing, 47*(6), 656–663.

Dahlen, H., Schmied, V., Downe, S., Tracy, S., Dowling, H., Upton, A., … & de Jonge, A. (2010). Facilitating physiological birth positioning in three different birth settings: an exploration into facilitators and inhibitors. *Journal of Paediatrics and Child Health, 46*(Suppl.1), 57–96.

Davis, H., & Day, C. (2010). *Working in Partnership with Parents.* London: Pearson.

Davis Floyd, R. (1997). *Childbirth and Authoritative Knowledge: Cross-cultural Perspectives.* Berkeley, CA: University of California Press.

Dreyfus, H., & Rabinow, P. (1983). *Michel Foucault. Beyond Structuralism and Hermeneutics,* 2nd edition. Chicago, IL: University of Chicago Press.

Emerson, R. (2009). Ethonography interaction and ordinary trouble. *Ethnography,* 10, 535–548.

Fahy, K.M., & Parratt, J.A. (2006). Birth territory: a theory for midwifery practice. *Women and Birth,* 19(2), 45–50.

Foucault, M. (1977). *Discipline and Punish. The Birth of the Prison* (translated by Alan Sheridan). London: Penguin.

Greenhalgh, T. and Sietsewieringa, S. (2011) Is it time to drop the 'knowledge translation' metaphor? A critical literature review, *Journal of the Royal Society of Medicine,* 104(12), 501–509.

Greenhalgh, Trisha, Robert, Glenn, Macfarlane, Fraser, Bate, Paul, & Kyriakidou, Olivia. (2004). Diffusion of innovations in service organizations: systematic review and recommendations. *Milbank Quarterly,* 82(4), 581–629.

Gupta, J.K., Hofmeyr, G.J., & Shehmar, M. (2012). Position in the second stage of labour for women without epidural anaesthesia. *Cochrane Database of Systematic Reviews.* http://onlinelibrary.wiley.com/doi/10.1002/14651858.CD002006.pub3/abstract

Hammersley, M. & Atkinson, P. (2007) *Ethnography: Principles in Practice,* 3rd edition, London: Routlege.

Harrison, A. (2011). Using 'observations of care' in nursing research: a discussion of methodological issues. *Journal of Research in Nursing,* 16(4), 377–387.

Harrison, S. (2002). New Labour, modernisation and the medical labour process. *Journal of Social Policy,* 31(3), 465–485.

Harvey, Gill, Loftus-Hills, Alison, Rycroft-Malone, Jo, Titchen, Angie, Kitson, Alison, McCormack, Brendan, & Seers, Kate. (2002). Getting evidence into practice: the role and function of facilitation. *Journal of Advanced Nursing,* 37(6), 577–588.

Hopwood, N., Fowler, C., Lee, A., Rossiter, C., & Bigsby, M. (2013). Understanding partnership practice in child and family nursing through the concept of practice architectures. *Nursing Inquiry,* 20(3), 199–210.

Jordan, B. (1992). *Birth in Four Culturees.* Long Grove, IL: Waveland Press.

Katz Rothman, B. (1989). *Recreating Motherhood: Ideology and Technology in a Patriarchal Society.* New York: W.W. Norton.

Kitson, A.L. (2009). The need for systems change: reflections on knowledge translation and organizational change. *Journal of Advanced Nursing,* 65(1), 217–228.

Lawrence, A., Lewis, L., Hofmeyr, G.J., and Styles, C. (2013) Maternal positions and mobility during first stage labour. *Cochrane Database of Systematic Reviews.* http://onlinelibrary.wiley.com/doi/10.1002/14651858.CD003934.pub4/abstract

Lupton, D. (1995). *The Imperative of Health: Public Health and The Regulated Body.* London: Sage.

Marcellus, L. (2005). The ethics of relation: public health nurses and child protection clients. *Journal of Advanced Nursing,* 51(4), 414–420.

McInnes, R.J., & Chambers, J.A. (2008). Supporting breastfeeding mothers: qualitative synthesis. *Journal of Advanced Nursing,* 62(4), 407–427.

National Health and Medical Research Council. (2003). *National Health and Medical Research Council Strategic Plan 2003–2006.* Canberra: NHMRC.

Noblit, G.W., & Hare, R.D. (1988). *Meta-ethnography: Synthesising Qualitative Studies.* Newbury Park, CA: Sage.

NSW Health. (2009). *NSW Health, Families NSW: Supporting Families Early Package.* North Sydney, NSW: NSW Dept of Health, 2009.

Peckover, S. (2003). Health visitors' understandings of domestic violence. *Journal of Advanced Nursing,* 44(2), 200–208.

Peterson, A., & Bunton, R. (1997). *Foucault, Health and Medicine.* London: Routledge.

Priddis, H., Dahlen, H., & Schmied, V. (2011). Juggling instinct and fear: an ethnographic study of facilitators and inhibitors of physiological birth positioning in two different birth settings. *International Journal of Childbirth,* 1(4), 227–241.

Priddis, H., Dahlen, H., & Schmied, V. (2012). What are the facilitators, inhibitors, and implications of birth positioning? A review of the literature. *Women and Birth,* 25(2), 100–106.

Renfrew, M.J., McCormick, F.M., Wade, A., Quinn, B., & Dowswell, T. (2012). Support for healthy breastfeeding mothers with healthy term babies. *Cochrane Database Of Systematic Reviews.* http://onlinelibrary.wiley.com/doi/10.1002/14651858.CD001141.pub4/abstract#content

Renfrew, M.J., McFadden, A., Bastos, M.H., Campbell, J., Channon, A.A., Cheung, N.F., … & Declercq, E. (2014). Midwifery and quality care: findings from a new evidence-informed framework for maternal and newborn care. *The Lancet,* 384(9948), 1129–1145.

Roche, B., Cowley, S., Salt, N., Scammell, A., Malone, M., Savile, P., … & Fitzpatrick, S. (2005). Reassurance or judgement? Parents' views on the delivery of child health surveillance programmes. *Family Practice,* 22(5), 507–512.

Rollans, M., Schmied, V., Kemp, L., & Meade, T. (2013a). Digging over that old ground: an Australian perspective of women's experience of psychosocial assessment and depression screening in pregnancy and following birth. *BMC Women's Health,* 13(1).

Rollans, M., Schmied, V., Kemp, L., & Meade, T. (2013b). Negotiating policy in practice: child and family health nurses' approach to the process of postnatal psychosocial assessment. *BMC Health Services Research,* 13(1).

Rollans, M., Schmied, V., Kemp, L., & Meade, T. (2013c). 'We just ask some questions…' the process of antenatal psychosocial assessment by midwives. *Midwifery,* 29(8), 935–942.

Sackett, D. (1997). Evidence-based medicine. *Seminars in Perinatology,* 21(1), 3–5.

Sackett, D.L., Rosenberg, W., Muir Gray, J.A., Haynes, R. Brian, & Richardson, W. Scott. (1996). Evidence based medicine: what it is and what it isn't – it's about integrating individual clinical expertise and the best external evidence. *BMJ: British Medical Journal,* 312(7023), 71–72. doi: 10.2307/29730277

Sarup, M. (1989). *An Introductory Guide to Post-structuralism and Postmodernism.* Athens, GA: University of Georgia Press.

Scamell, Mandie. (2011). The swan effect in midwifery talk and practice: a tension between normality and the language of risk. *Sociology of Health & Illness,* 33(7), 987–1001.

Schmied, V., Beake, S., Sheehan, A., McCourt, C., & Dykes, F. (2011). Women's experiences of breastfeeding support: a metasynthesis. *Birth,* 38, (1), 49–60.

Smeets, Wim, Gribnau, Frank, & van der Ven, Johannes. (2011). Quality assurance and spiritual care. *Journal of Empirical Theology,* 24(1), 80–121.

ten Hoope-Bender P., de Bernis L., Campbell J., Downe S., Fauveau V., Fogstad H., … & Van Lerberghe W. (2014). Improvement of maternal and newborn health through midwifery. *The Lancet,* 384(9949), 1226–1235.

Wilson, H.V. (2001). Power and partnership: a critical analysis of the surveillance discourses of child health nurses. *Journal of Advanced Nursing,* 36(2), 294–301.

6

CROSS-NATIONAL ETHNOGRAPHY IN NEONATAL INTENSIVE CARE UNITS

Renée Flacking and Fiona Dykes

In this chapter, we describe our experiences of conducting comparative ethnographic research in a highly medicalised setting, the neonatal intensive care unit (NICU) in Sweden and England. We start by presenting the rationale for conducting our cross-national ethnographic study, followed by briefly describing how the study was conducted. We then discuss key challenges throughout the planning, undertaking the research and the data analysis.

The rationale for conducting a cross-national comparative ethnographic study on feeding in preterm babies

Regardless of cultural setting, the birth of a preterm baby generates a situation in which the affected individuals are highly vulnerable and the mother–baby relationship is placed under pressure as the maternal role begins and develops within a highly medicalised and unfamiliar setting (Flacking et al., 2012). Preterm babies are immature in their development and unlike term babies often cannot be fully fed by breast or bottle from birth. Instead, mothers and babies experience a varying and sometimes long transition period from tube feeding to oral feeding, during which the mothers cannot take full responsibility for their babies' nutrition and survival in the way that parents of healthy babies born at term are usually able to do. Unfortunately, in many NICUs, this transitional feeding process has been, and still is, regulated by a diverse range of non-evidence-based guidelines and care routines. Examples include: the baby should be of a certain gestational age for breastfeeding to be initiated (Reyna et al., 2006); the baby should tolerate full oral feeds before initiating breastfeeding (Callen et al., 2005); the baby should be weighed before and after breastfeeding (test-weighing) in order to assess the milk intake (Meier et al.,

1996). Most research in the area of breastfeeding in preterm babies has focused on explanatory factors for weaning after a short breastfeeding period and thus attention has been paid to ways to optimise the transitional process in terms of milk intake. Few attempts have been made to assess parental perceptions of these care routines and the effects of these care routines on the breastfeeding duration (McInnes & Chambers, 2008). The transitional process is thus not only regulated by a diversity of non-evidence-based guidelines and care routines but also turned into a technical process with breastfeeding being seen as a 'product' and not part of a relational interplay. Previous studies by Flacking and colleagues (2006; 2007) have described breastfeeding as relational and integral to the process of becoming a mother. Findings from these Swedish studies indicated the importance of the interpersonal interplay between the mother and the baby/father/staff and of the public environment and care routines. The findings showed that the experience of separation, institutional authority, emotional exhaustion and the disregard for breastfeeding as a relational interplay, comprised major hindrances to experiencing breastfeeding as a mutual pleasure. Hence, mothers described their experiences of breastfeeding in a NICU as being at a 'training camp' and as dutiful and a task. Such experiences may result in earlier weaning from breastfeeding but, on the other hand depending on the culture, may lead to sustained breastfeeding due to the norm that a 'good mum breastfeeds'. Some of the key concepts and findings discovered in the previous work by Flacking and colleagues were inevitably very culturally specific, i.e. related to the public and cultural conditions in Sweden. For this reason, we wanted to conduct a more in-depth, cross-cultural study to understand the influence of differing cultures on mothers' experiences of breastfeeding their preterm baby in a NICU. The aim of our cross-national ethnographic study was therefore to explore breastfeeding/feeding and relationality in mothers of preterm babies at neonatal units in Sweden and England.

Epistemology and theoretical perspectives

The epistemology underpinning our ethnographic research stems from social constructionism, which, as Crotty (1998) describes, is the view that knowledge and hence reality, is constructed in and out of social interaction and is developed and conveyed within a particular social context. Social constructionism emphasises that the generation of meaning is always social and related to cultural contexts (Crotty, 1998).

The theoretical perspective that we applied to this research stemmed from the ecological perspective summarised by McLaren and Hawe (2005). This highlights the interdependence and interplay between people and their environments – with a concern to understand and take account of physical, social, cultural, and historical contexts as well as attributes and behaviours of people. It also shifts the focus away from reductionism and linear causality towards a more holistic outlook that appreciates and embraces complexity.

This perspective will be used to identify the macro (national/societal), meso (community) and micro (family/individual) issues with regard to our research question. The macro perspective (national/societal) in our study relates to the social, economic and health policy contexts. The meso perspective relates to the local NICU environments to include the organisation of care staffing structures and the design of these specific health care environments. The micro perspective relates to individual experiences within the specific NICUs.

Wrede et al. (2006) make the case for a cross-cultural comparison in health research that takes the meso level as its starting point. That includes the design of health care organisations, professional groups and other health-related organisations. They argue that most comparative health care research remains at the macro level with insufficient consideration of the social and cultural contexts. Wrede et al. (2006) conducted cross-national research comparing maternity care in eight high-income European and North American countries. This involved engaging researchers with in-depth knowledge of the culture and context of each country, thus avoiding the risk of making one set of assumptions common to all countries. They referred to this as the decentred approach to cross-national research. Wrede et al. (2006) recommend three central components utilised in the analysis: firstly an avoidance of using one homogenous set of assumptions for assessing the differences in maternity care; secondly, treating the macro, meso and micro levels of analysis as related but analytically separate; and third, "integration of culture as a significant dimension of analysis so that organisations, rules, routines, procedures and assumptions are regarded as cultural products that shape and are shaped by the distinctive milieu of each country" (Wrede et al., 2006, p. 2993).

Key differences between Sweden and England

Macro level

Sweden has long been thought of as a country that is fairly homogenous in terms of the income of its inhabitants with very low levels of social deprivation. This is still somewhat true as Sweden is one of the nine most 'equal' countries within the Organisation for Economic Co-operation and Development (OECD), despite the fact that the increase in inequality was the largest among all OECD countries between 1985 and the late 2000s. England has a much higher level of income inequality compared with Sweden. Sweden is the highest spender on public services such as health and care among the OECD countries (Organisation for Economic Co-operation and Development, 2011). Public spending on family benefits includes parental financial benefit for 13 months with 80 per cent of the income and three months with 180 SEK/day. In 2011, about 76 per cent of the days were claimed by mothers and 23 per cent by fathers (Swedish Social Insurance Agency, 2012). Additional parental benefits are 10 days of paternity leave in connection with the baby's birth and 120 days of temporary parental benefit per child and year, which enables parents to stay home from work when their children are sick. These legislations are considered to be supportive for a long duration of breastfeeding (Galtry, 2003). In England the Statutory Maternity Pay is paid for up to 39 weeks. For the first six weeks the mother gets 90 per cent of the average weekly earnings. For the following 33 weeks the mother gets £138 or 90 per cent of the average weekly earnings (whichever is lower).

In Sweden, cost-free perinatal care reaches almost all mothers, and 93 per cent of primiparous women attend childbirth and parenthood education classes (Fabian et al., 2004). Health care for children is cost-free, with a few exceptions, and includes regular visits to child health centres, which nearly all families attend. This public service is responsible for health promotion as well as health surveillance of babies from birth until school age, and this enables assessment of breastfeeding up to one year of baby age. In England, health care is also cost-free via the National Health Service as has been described for Sweden.

In 2012, 96 per cent of all Swedish babies were being breastfed at one week of age, 64 per cent at six months and 18 per cent at one year of age (National Board of Health and Welfare, 2014). In 2010, 69 per cent of all English babies were being breastfed at one week of age and 34 per cent at six months (McAndrew et al., 2012). The differences in breastfeeding rates between Sweden and England reflect two quite contrasting infant and young child feeding cultures.

Meso level

Institutional culture has been described as a series of layers with shared behavioural expectations and norms representing an outer, conscious layer, and values and assumptions representing an inner, less conscious layer (Glisson & Green, 2005). Whilst the 'inner', tacit part is important to understand, there is evidence to suggest that culture is expressed and transmitted through 'visible' shared behavioural expectations and norms rather than through 'invisible' values or assumptions (Glisson & Green, 2005). It is therefore argued that individuals may be compliant with behavioural norms and expectations, without necessarily being consciously aware of the underpinning values and beliefs that direct their day-to-day practice (Glisson & Green, 2005).

An example of difference at the meso level relates to the design of NICUs' relates to the design of NICUs. A survey conducted in Europe showed that 100 per cent of the included units in Sweden and 11 per cent of those in the UK had reclining chairs near babies' cots, and beds for the parents were provided in 100 per cent of the Swedish units and 77 per cent of the UK units (Greisen et al., 2009). Another cultural difference between NICUs relates to parental visiting opportunities. In the UK, many units do not allow parents to be present during medical ward rounds, nursing shift handovers and 'quiet periods' (Hamilton & Redshaw, 2009). In our study there were four NICUs. In one unit parents could stay during the intensive care phase in a parental bed next to the incubator in a room shared with up to three other babies/families but with screens in between. After the intensive care phase, for example when ventilation was no longer required, the baby was transferred with the parent(s) to a single room, in which the whole family (including siblings) could stay for the remaing part of the hospital stay. Infants who needed less intensive care (e.g. no ventilation) were transferred with the parent, straight after delivery, to their own room, where they stayed for the entire hospital stay. In two of the units there were reclining or comfortable chairs by most incubators or cots, and in both units there were designated rooms for parents (five and four respectively) that were used as a single room for the family or shared between two mothers. In one of the units there were fewer comfortable chairs and very few rooms that parents could stay in.

Micro level

Clearly the experiences of parents relates directly and indirectly to the macro and meso level factors. These experiences are not referred to here but are described in detail in our paper "'Being in a womb' or 'playing musical chairs': the impact of place and space on infant feeding in NICUs" (Flacking & Dykes, 2013). The paper focuses specifically upon the impact of space and place on the experiences of parents and staff. When space and place generates a separation between mother and baby, it may contribute towards the mother feeling unimportant and reduce her status to that of a visitor. When the place is constructed so that a mother has a sense of ownership of place/space this in turn helps to facilitate her in feeling ownership of her own body and her baby and supports her in feeling important as a mother and as a person. Thus, when space and place are designed so that the mother's own emotional and physical needs are met and where she can be 'present' emotionally it facilitates an attunement in which there is a shared awareness and a balance between the mother and her baby.

Cross-national ethnography

Very few studies have been performed in the medical setting with a cross-national ethnographic design. Some studies have been described as 'ethnographic' – although there is no observation conducted, merely interviews. However, conducting interviews may at the same time be observations. While interviewing or having an informal conversation the participants can be observed in an informal and natural setting. Hence, in-depth interviews can be designed to engage participants in their own environment. An example of this was a study conducted by Kingman and colleagues (2014) who undertook an ethnographic study in seven countries with the aim of understanding pulmonary hypertension from the patient's perspective. The research aims and methodology were developed collaboratively with some input from an international, multidisciplinary advisory group. The researchers (all native speakers of the local language in the country where the research took place) filmed and observed patients in their home for up to six hours. The researchers had a loose discussion guide but adjusted it to whatever the patient chose to do on the day of the visit. Data were supplemented with diaries in which the patients wrote about their perspective of the illness and included four tasks titled: *my perfect day*, *how my treatment makes me feel*, *letter to my doctor* and *if my illness was a person*. All data was translated into English and after the analysis sessions a 45 min ethnographic film was then produced from each country. In addition, an hour-long international film highlighting the key findings was produced.

Our cross-national, comparative study in NICUs in Sweden and England involved 11 months of participant observation of activities on the NICUs, with particular reference to interactions between unit staff, mothers, fathers and their babies related to baby feeding. Observations were made during day and night shifts over a period of three months in Sweden, six months in England and then two further months in Sweden by Renée who travelled back and forth between the two units in each country. The observations were made by sitting in those rooms where parents, their babies, and staff spent most of their time and were supplemented by interviews relating to what had been observed. During the observations, field notes were taken and where possible interviews were recorded using a digital tape recorder. A nine-dimension framework for data collection (Spradley, 1980) was used initially. Later on, more focused observations were made in order to answer the research questions and elicit more specific aspects. In total, 600 hours of fieldwork were performed, of which 300 hours were direct observations and interviews. In Sweden, 112 observations/interviews were made on parents, of which 38 included both the mother and father. In England, 57 observations/interviews were made on parents, of which 11 included both the mother and father. In Sweden, 108 hours of observations and 54 hours of interviews (a total of 59 interviews, range 10–120 minutes, mean 55 minutes) were conducted. In England, 102 hours of observations and 42 hours of interviews (a total of 46 interviews, range 10–120 minutes, mean 55 minutes) were conducted.

Key challenges

Conducting ethnography in hospital

For centuries ethnography was rarely undertaken in hospitals. Van der Geest and Finkler (2004) propose that the reason for this was that hospitals were familiar settings to many potential researchers. At first glance hospitals may look strikingly similar; the organisation of care with separate units, long corridors, staff uniforms and medical equipment. In many ways, NICUs worldwide have important medical similarities. They may use the same ventilators, observational equipment and the same medicines, regardless of whether it is a NICU in Hong Kong, Australia or Sweden. In neonatal care and in NICUs medical care and technology have improved tremendously in the last decade, to the extent that we can now save babies born in the 22nd gestational week (Fellman et al., 2009). However, several studies and benchmarking projects have shown that the quality of neonatal care differs between and within countries in Europe on major outcomes such as mortality and neonatal complications of prematurity (Draper et al., 2009; Serenius et al., 2014). Even more marked differences are found in outcomes such as breastfeeding rates (Bonet et al., 2011). The 'culture' of neonatal units, for example the provision of neonatal care and parental involvement, may reflect and reinforce social processes to such an extent that it actually has an impact on morbidity and mortality. By using ethnography in hospitals we gain a deeper understanding of 'what happens' and 'why it happens' in and between units. Van der Geest and Finkler state that "biomedicine, and the hospital as its foremost institution is a domain where the core values and beliefs of a culture come into view" (2004, p. 1996).

Before we undertook our study we anticipated that there would be large differences between England and Sweden in terms of neonatal care and parental involvement and this was indeed the case. The major difference was parental presence. After the first few months of the study in Sweden where parents were present most of the day and night, the contrast to the English neonatal units was apparent. In one of Renée's first field notes from England, she noted: "To be able to look at relationality there needs to be parents here to observe but there aren't. Where are they? How can I find them?" This 'absence' of parents was striking for someone coming from the Swedish context and although parents *were* present in the English units there was a vast difference that probably reflects the different standards of maternity leave and benefits. What we expected to a lesser extent were the differences we observed within the countries (i.e. between the two units in each country). This was especially evident in England, where our observations may reflect a more diverse society with large socioeconomic disparities. Before the project started we visited the units and were shown around. At the first visit, after about 10 minutes, Renée saw a person coming around with a trolley with coffee, tea and chocolate biscuits for parents and staff. How very English! The person who showed us around described the unit's 'policy' – that parents should be seen as the baby's primary caregiver at all times. We were therefore not let into any rooms where there were babies until the parents consented. If they did not or if they were not present we had to stay outside the room. As a contrast, in the other English unit there was a poster up on the wall describing four benefits of rooming in (e.g. "helps to promote baby-led feeding" and "baby will learn to recognise mum"). This poster could be seen as a display of a 'core value'. The problem was that there were only one or two rooms available for rooming in and they were mostly used during the last 24–48 hours before discharge and hence not for what was communicated through the poster. These examples show the relationship between 'core values' and how integrated they can be or not be in care and practice. When there is a connection between what we 'say' and what we 'do' care becomes comprehensible but when there is no link it becomes disruptive and we start to question ourselves or the care. Furthermore, these examples may also indicate 'cultures' being person-centred versus institutionalised. A subsequent question is whether a person-centred approach is more common in an area populated by higher earners and an institutionalised approach more common in a socially deprived area, as they were in our study.

There has been an increase of ethnographic studies conducted in hospitals, some of which were undertaken within NICUs (see for example Cricco-Lizza, 2011; 2014; Einarsdottir, 2012). One reason for this increase might be that there is a more open attitude towards ethnography and that the findings are valuable for the understanding and development of care. However, gatekeepers and staff may be reluctant to allow observers to enter their unit and be observed. Before we commenced our study, we identified several possible NICUs in Sweden and England. Some were excluded because of travelling distance, others because they were too alike, and a few because of less positive gatekeepers. When an ethnographic study is to be undertaken you do not need people who are overwhelmingly positive but you do need people who can 'open the doors', that can introduce the study in a positive way and who you can communicate with if problems arise. Therefore it is very important to choose units/wards where the gatekeepers can be of assistance and not a hindrance.

Reflexivity

Reflexivity is central to effective cross-national comparative work. As stated, our research was underpinned by a social constructionist perspective so it was particularly important that we were aware of our own cultural lenses through which we saw the world. These were inevitably quite different as Renée was enculturated in Sweden and Fiona in England. Furthermore, Renée had worked in a NICU for more than 10 years. Ideas about how concepts are related to explain a certain phenomenon are rooted in one's own disciplinary perspective and this view of the world is determined by the concepts the researcher values. Whilst it has to be acknowledged that any level of participant observation involves the researcher interacting with and affecting the environment in which s/he is researching, it is important to be reflexive about this during the entire research process to include data collection, analysis and reporting.

Before we commenced our study we were fully aware of the challenge of 'familiarity' and sought ways to keep reflexive minds. When conducting an ethnographic study participant informed interpretations are written down along with the observed behaviours. Renée continuously recorded feelings, ideas and thoughts about the phenomena we studied in a field journal. She also noted useful discussions with other Swedish and English researchers, and Fiona in particular. During the discussions, Renée presented findings, interpretations and ideas while Fiona's task was to question and even challenge Renée's interpretations in relation to her personal values and ideas. By having such discussions, we trained our minds to be more critical and question our own beliefs and values and over time we also could identify 'personal values' more easily.

Ethical aspects

Participant observation raises challenging ethical questions. Doing a cross-national ethnographic study raises even more questions. We will highlight three important aspects to reflect on before undertaking cross-national ethnographic studies or ethnographic research into neonatal intensive care.

The process for ethical clearance in different countries

In most research ethical approval from an ethical board (e.g. university, health service, regional or national) is needed before commencing a study. When we are familiar with our own context we usually 'know' how to go about it; what needs to be submitted, to whom, time between submission and approval, and potential costs. As the process might look very different in different countries, as was the case in our study, it is wise to do some research into this early on in the process. Sweden has a fairly straightforward ethical vetting (i.e. reviewing and approving research proposals regarding their ethics). The ethical vetting is conducted by one of six regional boards (situated at six universities in Sweden). The regional boards are independent authorities responsible for their own geographically defined catchment area. Within each regional board there is one section whose purpose is to vet cases within the field of medical science (medicine, pharmacology, odontology, the science of health care and clinical psychology). The sections have a number of highly qualified scientific members and also representatives from the general public. All members and their substitutes are appointed by the government. The sections have meetings regularly (about 1–2 times/month), which means that it usually takes 4–6 weeks to get an approval after the proposal has been submitted. There is a cost involved, currently the fee is 5.000 SEK for a single-site study and 16.000 SEK for a multi-centre study. In England, ethical vetting may take considerably longer as the application has to be processed thoroughly by the National Health Service Research Ethics Committee, University Ethics Committees and relevant Research and Development committees at each research site. This process may take up to six months to complete.

Informed consent in neonatal intensive care

Our study included both staff and parents of preterm babies. Information about the study was presented to the staff before commencing the study at specific staff meetings. All staff working at each unit were also given written information about the study and if they agreed to participate a signed consent form was given to Renée. Staff were assured that they were free to withdraw at any time and at certain times. Two staff did not want to be observed at all, one of whom was experiencing personal problems at that time. On a few occasions, staff clearly signalled that they did not want to be observed through body language or by verbally saying "today I'm a bit stressed out so maybe not today…?", and were thus not observed that day.

Mothers and fathers were given oral and written information about the study a day or so after the baby was admitted to the unit. In those cases where the baby was critically ill, information was given when he/she was stabilised. 'Critically ill' is an ambiguous concept and hence much consideration and empathy were required. Although Renée or staff members did not consider the baby to be 'critically ill', parents may have done so. Therefore, Renée tried to put herself into 'the shoes of the parent' and mostly when there was a slight reason to believe that parents experienced their baby as 'critically ill', Renée refrained from observing.

All information about the study was given to the mothers and fathers by Renée to avoid a conflict of interest. The reason why the staff did not provide information and obtain written consent was that there might have been a coercive element to it, in that mothers and fathers might endeavour to please the staff. Renée approached the mother/father and asked if it might be possible to talk to her/him about the study. If they agreed to the conversation, the study was explained verbally and by written information. The mothers and fathers were invited to read about the study and think about participating for 24 hours. After a day, the researcher approached them again and asked if they had any further questions and obtained written consent from those agreeing to participate. This time period of 24 hours enabled parents to discuss and ponder on their participation. Parents who agreed to participate signed a consent form. Mothers and fathers were told they were free to withdraw at any time. This was communicated at the beginning and throughout the field studies. It was of particular importance to avoid intruding upon mothers' and fathers' privacy and space. Thus, before the start of each 'shift', the mothers and fathers who had initially consented to participate were asked again if they were willing to be observed/interviewed. However, sometimes even asking was too much. Having a preterm baby in a neonatal unit is like being on an emotional roller-coaster (Flacking et al., 2006; 2007). Hence, Renée had to be sensitive to body language. This included noting expressions such as fatigue, sadness or anger and responding by not asking the parent if it was ok to make observations or carefully concluding an interview or an observation.

An ethical dilemma was that there were often several parents in the same room, some of whom were asked to participate and some were not because of the inclusion criteria of prematurity. Participants not selected may have felt excluded or not interesting enough. It was made clear to non-participants that they had not been approached because they had a term baby and that observations only related to those who had provided a consent form.

Cultural norms

Cultural norms are shared, sanctioned, and integrated systems of beliefs and practices that characterise a cultural group, such as a NICU. A norm is hence an acceptable and expected way of behaving in any given social situation. A behaviour, or rather an 'unacceptable behaviour', becomes an ethical issue when the researcher observes or is informed about something that may cause harm, illness, ill-being, damage or put someone at risk. Implementing evidence into practice is an urgent global issue (World Health Organization, 2006). A widely cited report claims that 30–40 per cent of all patients do not receive health care based on current relevant knowledge and the implementation of research into clinical practice continues to be a major challenge for researchers and health care professionals (Grimshaw et al., 2006; Grol & Grimshaw, 2003; Wallin, 2009). So where do we, as ethnographic researchers, draw the line for 'acceptable behaviour and actions'? Who decides what an unacceptable behaviour/action is? Who has the responsibility and accountability?

In our study, we observed that certain parental/staff behaviours and actions were acceptable in one unit or in one country but not in other units/countries, according to informal/formal 'rules' or norms. We will present two quite different examples of cultural norms that were accepted in one unit but not in other units. First, an example of noise. In three of the units, staff spoke in a low voice, alarms were quickly muted and there was an overall silence in the units. In all these three units, 'SoundEars' were mounted to the wall. The 'SoundEar' was intended to indicate noise level (40 dB to 115 dB) in an easy to understand manner (green, yellow and red light), and could omit a warning whenever the noise level got too high, which rarely happened during observations. In the fourth unit, 'SoundEars' were also fixed to the wall but turned off, either completely (no light of green, yellow or red) or partially (lights indicated the volume but the warning sound when red was muted). In this unit the noise was often prominent. In some rooms the radio was on quite loudly with music playing and commercial interruptions. In other rooms, the sound from monitors was overpowering. There is quite good evidence documenting the damaging effects of noise on the preterm infant's development. A noisy environment creates negative physiologic responses in the infant (e.g. apnoea, bradycardia). Preterm infants exposed to prolonged high noise levels are also at increased risk for abnormal brain and sensory development (Hassanein et al., 2013; Vandenberg, 2007). Thus, the lack of efforts to minimise the harmful effects of the environment became an ethical issue for us when conducting the study.

The second example concerned feeding. In one of the units babies were bottle fed by staff in, from Renée's point of view, a very 'unusual position'. Staff held the babies sitting sideways (i.e. baby's side towards staff's stomach) far out on the person's lap in a position mediated by the staff holding the baby's neck in a firm grip. From the perspective of developmental care and support, it was felt that these babies lacked the physical support they needed in order to feel well and coordinate breathing and swallowing in their own pace. When staff were asked about this they referred to their own personal preferences (e.g. "I like to feed this way" or "I have a better control") or that the baby did not fall asleep when being fed this way. This behaviour was considered 'acceptable' in the unit but not observed nor 'acceptable' in the three other units. When discovering this phenomena and the rationale for the behaviour we discussed it with one of the supervisors of midwives from the maternity unit. We concluded that this practice would not be seen as misconduct but a poor way to care for babies during feeding. Thus, whilst it was not considered 'best practice' it was not considered malpractice. Furthermore, Renée was there in her capacity as a researcher in order to observe and not to change practice on site at the time.

Language

It is difficult to understand and to describe human emotions across both cultures and languages, yet we do. Emotions are not only expressed through spoken words, but also through facial and bodily expressions, which are more universal than words. Wierzbicka states: "the emotional language of the face is to a considerable extent universal, and not dependent on language-specific vocabulary of emotions" (2009, p. 7). Hence, facial expressions help us to understand the meaning of words that are used to describe an emotion.

However, when writing we use words and much of the scientific literature is written in the English language. Non-native English-speaking people adapt and translate their study findings into English, either by a translator or by having a qualified language reviewer that you may work closely with to find the 'right' words. English words and expressions are not universal concepts. English words are English words. There may be particular English words that need sentences in another language to describe the meaning or, vice versa, words that are very difficult to translate into English. Furthermore, languages are dynamic in that new words are invented and used and some go out of fashion. A word can used by a certain group and mean something, whilst for another group it means something completely different. A word can also have different meanings but be acknowledged as such by all citizens speaking the language. For example, the Swedish word 'gift' means both 'poison' and 'married' but the meaning is generally easy to understand because of the context.

The researcher who did all the observations and interviews, Renée, was a native-Swedish speaker. She had lived in the US for a year, she had written papers and her thesis in English and she had spent a lot of time in the UK before commencing the study. Hence, she spoke more than good-enough English to communicate. However, words became so much more than just words during the study. As humans we use words to describe how we think and feel which can be seen as representations of emotions. Words that are familiar to us are taken for granted. When trying to understand the meaning behind the words in another language you discover that one should be conscientious in one's own language.

The study started out in Sweden for three months and then moved on to England for six months. Early on in the English part of our study the word 'cuddle' was used. It was a word that appeared quite often when parents talked about being close to the babies. It seemed to be an important phenomenon but the word was unfamiliar to Renée. Intrigued about the meaning and the emotions related to the concept, parents and staff were asked to explain what it meant. But most parents and staff struggled when trying to explain such a 'normal' concept used in everyday language. Most participants agreed that it was 'more than a hug'. It was a word that carried a "culture-specific emotional script" (Wierzbicka, 2009, p. 13). Finally, Renée asked a close friend and research colleague, Kenny, who explained it beautifully:

> A cuddle is an extended hug, more warmth and more affection. Gentle and soothing. It's more than a hug and it can be applied to a baby in a way that a hug couldn't. You can't hug a baby… It can also apply to any situation where you hug… but softer. You greet people with a hug. You wouldn't say, 'give them a cuddle'. A hug has more empathy and comfort. A lot of the time it's for reassurance, to feel supported. It's taking someone in your arms.

So, initially, what might have been considered a huge problem, not being native-English, became enriching. After the six months in England, an additional two months were conducted in Sweden. The reason for that was not to explore words and meanings *per se* but nevertheless it became an in-depth exploration of culturally specific concepts.

Wild and colleagues (2005) have presented a set of principles of good practice in the translation and cultural adaption of patient-reported outcomes. The steps in the translation process as suggested by Wild et al. (2005) are: 1) preparation, 2) forward translation, 3) reconciliation, 4) back translation, 5) back translation review, 6) harmonisation, 7) cognitive debriefing, 8) review of cognitive debriefing, 9) proofreading and 10) final report. Although the rationale, and partly the process, for translation are different depending on what we aim to achieve, these steps are highly relevant when translating distinctive and culturally important concepts. By using steps such as reconciliation, harmonisation and cognitive debriefing we can discuss, explain and detect discrepancies between languages and words, test alternatives and assess if the translation is cognitively equivalent and comprehensible. Maybe more than one word is needed to describe what an English 'cuddle' is?

Level of participation – sitting in a corner

As referred to in Chapter 1, Spradley (1980) refers to four levels of participation ranging from 'low' engagement to 'high' (p. 58). We chose a 'moderate' level of participation (Spradley, 1980) involving a balance between observation and participation, meaning that Renée could, when relevant, answer simple questions, or assist mothers by, for example, fetching things. In one of the units Renée was dressed like any member of staff, because of the acknowledged risk of infections. In three of the units, she was dressed as a non-staff member from the waist down and had a staff shirt on. The rationale for being dressed partly as a member of staff was (1) because of the risk for spreading infections but also (2) to distinguish oneself from the staff *and* from the parents. By choosing a middle option Renée was not seen as staff by parents but also not as 'an intruder' that could be seen as a potential threat. In all units Renée had an identification badge which made it clear that she was a 'Researcher'.

One of the challenges experienced while undertaking our study was that 'rooms' may look very different and will hence influence how one, as a researcher, may be able to observe and interact with participants. In the research protocol we stated: "The observations will be made by the researcher sitting in those rooms where mothers, fathers, and their infants are. During the observations, field notes will be taken. The observations will be supplemented by interviews (short and informal conversations) that relate to what has been observed, with staff, mothers, and fathers, following observation." This worked well when the rooms were spacious, where there were a lot of people and much was happening. However, when mothers and fathers had a single room where they stayed, slept and cared for the baby, it became emotionally difficult to sit in a corner and observe. In those situations 'just observing' would have conveyed a message that parents were assessed and judged. Hence, a much more 'natural' approach was chosen in which Renée entered their room as a guest and where chatting became a vital part of the observations. By using 'chatting' as a method to be present in their room, realistic observations could be made of actions taking place. A potential threat to trustworthiness in ethnography stems from the 'Hawthorne effect'. As stated in Chapter 1, this relates to the effect of being studied upon those being studied with knowledge of the study possibly influencing behaviour. The participants may become more interested in the subject area or they may change their behaviour simply because someone (a researcher) is showing an interest in them (Parsons, 1974). However, mothers/fathers/staff who are being observed for a long time may habituate to the researcher's presence. Furthermore, the informants were very explicit in their views and did not seem to construct themselves to fulfil 'expected' norms or to please the researcher; the same was evident for staff. In addition, in line with a constructionist epistemology, one can recognise the researcher as part of the construction of the social situation.

Emotional management

How to cope with one's own emotions during a substantial time period of ethnographic research is rarely described but definitely important. Unlike other forms of qualitative research, the ethnographer participates in people's lives for months. Parents have shared their most inner thoughts, you have seen them struggle, you worry about the baby and the parents when critical events happen and you feel sad when you see sadness in people's eyes. Although Renée had worked as a neonatal nurse for years and had previously conducted qualitative work in NICUs, the magnitude of emotional turmoil was unexpected. The emotional struggle experienced was mainly related to two aspects.

'Your hands are tied behind your back'

The purpose of being an ethnographic researcher is to explore phenomena, not to help, assist or support participating parents or staff. The researcher knows that and the participants know that. The challenge is that a breach may occur between the cognitive evaluation of the ideal self in two differing roles, i.e. the kind, warm supporting nurse 'in me' and the impartial researcher who observes and reports. This self-evaluation gave rise to shame which emerged through an awareness of a deficiency or a feeling of not being good or good enough. Shame is often confused with guilt but they are considered to be two distinct emotions (Scheff, 1997). Guilt refers to behaviours where you have the feeling that you have done a 'bad thing' whilst shame is an "an experience that affects and is affected by the whole self", in which the self "stands revealed" (Lynd, 1958). The shame may arise while doing the observations or at the end of a session when you have the time to reflect. Hence, this shame is based on the evaluation of 'self' in the form of its imagined appearance to the parents/staff and the imagined judgement of that appearance by those participants. What arise are feelings of inadequacy that one can't help out or a feeling of failing due to withholding information/knowledge. When shame is denied, unacknowledged or hidden, it becomes disruptive (Lewis, 1971) and therefore it is of importance to communicate these emotions if they do arise. While conducting our study, feelings of helplessness, sadness and shame were communicated between Renée and Fiona as well as with other researchers. This helped emotionally and by having these discussions we could also view our data from a more in-depth emotional perspective. This emotional debriefing is crucial for the well-being of the researcher conducting ethnographic field work.

'Buried in data'

The amount of data gathered in an ethnographic study is often more than a 'handful'. In our study, observations and interviews were conducted almost every day. It is very easy to leave taped interviews and messy field notes after a day's work. It is suggested that "it is a grave error to let this work build up without regular reflection and review" (Hammersley & Atkinson, 2007, p. 151). Hence, all interviews were transcribed within a couple of days and field notes were written up as processed notes in Word documents the same day they were made. Data were organised chronologically and a matrix of all observations and interviews, including the codes of participating staff and parents, lengths of observation/interview etc. This matrix became a crucial facility, for finding data or selecting a specific family and analysing their process. Furthermore, all data had to be processed continuously as we utilised a grounded theory approach (Glaser, 1998). The analysis of data involved interpretation of the meanings, functions, and consequences of actions and institutional practices. Transcripts were initially coded to identify concepts in the data; these concepts were then grouped together into preliminary codes. During this phase of the coding, each incident was compared with other already identified concepts through observations and interviews (i.e. constant comparative method) and hence codes. Identified codes and their properties and dimensions constituted a continuously developing 'framework' for further observations/interviews. This description of how we conducted the study and analysed the data sounds straightforward. However, after 11 months of fieldwork, the magnitude of data is enormous and it was, and still is, an emotional challenge not to feel discouraged or helpless when writing papers. The only thing that helps is to get on with it!

Conclusion

There is a lack of research performed in the medical setting with a cross-national ethnographic design. With more in-depth, cross-cultural studies exploring the influences of different cultures on values, behaviours and practices we would stand on much better ground when designing interventions, evaluating their transferability and the potential for implementing 'successful' interventions. In this chapter we have presented the challenges we experienced whilst undertaking our cross-international ethnographic study. What we assume and anticipate when starting out a journey of explorations may be vastly different from what we encounter. Hence, some pre-research in terms of finding suitable sites with 'happy-enough' gatekeepers will be beneficial. It is also better to be a time-pessimist than a time-optimist, especially when applying for ethical clearance and time needed to analyse and write up the data. The importance of having a team involved cannot be over-emphasised. With a cross-national team of researchers, ideas, values, and beliefs can be discussed (to enhance reflexivity and reduce familiarity) and ethical aspects reflected and pondered on (to ensure that the best actions will be taken). Furthermore, the research team should provide a safe 'harbour' for those who are doing the observations and interviews; a team with whom emotions can be shared and acknowledged in a secure way.

References

Bonet, M., Blondel, B., Agostino, R., Combier, E., Maier, R.F., Cuttini, M. et al. (2011) Variations in breastfeeding rates for very preterm infants between regions and neonatal units in Europe: results from the MOSAIC cohort. *Archives of Disease in Childhood – Fetal Neonatal Edition* 96, 450–452.

Callen, J., Pinelli, J., Atkinson, S., & Saigal, S. (2005) Qualitative analysis of barriers to breastfeeding in very-low-birthweight infants in the hospital and postdischarge. *Advances in Neonatal Care* 5, 93–103.

Cricco-Lizza, R. (2011) Everyday nursing practice values in the NICU and their reflection on breastfeeding promotion. *Qualitative Health Research* 21, 399–409.

Cricco-Lizza, R. (2014) The need to nurse the nurse: emotional labor in neonatal intensive care. *Qualitative Health Research* 24, 615–628.

Crotty, M. (1998) *The Foundations of Social Research. Meaning and Perspective in the Research Process.* London: Sage Publications.

Draper, E.S., Zeitlin, J., Fenton, A.C., Weber, T., Gerrits, J., Martens, G. et al. (2009) Investigating the variations in survival rates for very preterm infants in 10 European regions: the MOSAIC birth cohort. *Archives of Disease in Childhood – Fetal Neonatal Edition* 94, F158–163.

Einarsdottir, J. (2012) Happiness in the neonatal intensive care unit: merits of ethnographic fieldwork. *International Journal of Qualitative Studies in Health and Well-being* 7, 1–9.

Fabian, H.M., Radestad, I.J., & Waldenstrom, U. (2004) Characteristics of Swedish women who do not attend childbirth and parenthood education classes during pregnancy. *Midwifery* 20, 226–235.

Fellman, V., Hellstrom-Westas, L., Norman, M., Westgren, M., Kallen, K., Lagercrantz, H. et al. (2009) One-year survival of extremely preterm infants after active perinatal care in Sweden. *JAMA* 301, 2225–2233.

Flacking, R., & Dykes, F. (2013) 'Being in a womb' or 'playing musical chairs': the impact of place and space on infant feeding in NICUs. *BMC Pregnancy Childbirth* 13, 179.

Flacking, R., Ewald, U., Nyqvist, K.H., & Starrin, B. (2006) Trustful bonds: a key to 'becoming a mother' and to reciprocal breastfeeding. Stories of mothers of very preterm infants at a neonatal unit. *Social Science & Medicine* 62, 70–80.

Flacking, R., Ewald, U., & Starrin, B. (2007) 'I wanted to do a good job': experiences of becoming a mother and breastfeeding in mothers of very preterm infants after discharge from a neonatal unit. *Social Science & Medicine* 64, 2405–2416.

Flacking, R., Lehtonen, L., Thomson, G., Axelin, A., Ahlqvist, S., Moran, V.H. et al. (2012) Closeness and separation in neonatal intensive care. *Acta Paediatrica* 101, 1032–1037.

Galtry, J. (2003) The impact on breastfeeding of labour market policy and practice in Ireland, Sweden, and the USA. *Social Science & Medicine* 57, 167–177.

Glaser, B. (1998) *Doing Grounded Theory: Issues and Discussions.* Mill Valley, CA: Sociology Press.

Glisson, C., & Green, P. (2005) The effects of organizational culture and climate on the access to mental health care in child welfare and juvenile justice systems. *Administration and Policy in Mental Health Services Research* 33, 433–448.

Greisen, G., Mirante, N., Haumont, D., Pierrat, V., Pallás-Alonso, C., Warren, I. et al. (2009) Parents, siblings and grandparents in the neonatal intensive care unit. A survey of policies in eight European countries. *Acta Paediatrica* 98, 1744–1750.

Grimshaw, J., Eccles, M., Thomas, R., MacLennan, G., Ramsay, C., Fraser, C. et al. (2006) Toward evidence-based quality improvement. Evidence (and its limitations) of the effectiveness of guideline dissemination and implementation strategies 1966–1998. *Journal of General Internal Medicine* 21 Suppl 2, S14–20.

Grol, R., & Grimshaw, J. (2003) From best evidence to best practice: effective implementation of change in patients' care. *Lancet* 362, 1225–1230.

Hamilton, K., & Redshaw, M. (2009) Developmental care in the UK: a developing initiative. *Acta Paediatrica* 98, 1738–1743.

Hammersley, M., & Atkinson, P. (2007) *Ethnography: Principles in Practice* (3rd edn). London: Routledge.

Hassanein, S.M., El Raggal, N.M., & Shalaby, A.A. (2013) Neonatal nursery noise: practice-based learning and improvement. *Journal of Maternal-Fetal & Neonatal Medicine* 26, 392–395.

Kingman, M., Hinzmann, B., Sweet, O., & Vachiery, J.L. (2014) Living with pulmonary hypertension: unique insights from an international ethnographic study. *BMJ Open* 4, e004735.

Lewis, H. (1971) *Shame and Guilt in Neurosis*. New York: International Universities Press.

Lynd, H. (1958) *On Shame and the Search for Identity*. New York: Science Editions.

McAndrew, F., Thompson, J., Fellows, L., Large, A., Speed, M., & Renfrew, M. (2012). Infant Feeding Survey 2010. London: The Information Centre for Health and Social Care and the UK Health Departments. http://www.hscic.gov.uk/catalogue/PUB08694/Infant-Feeding-Survey-2010-Consolidated-Report.pdf.

McInnes, R., & Chambers, J. (2008) Infants admitted to neonatal units – interventions to improve breastfeeding outcomes: a systematic review 1990–2007. *Maternal and Child Nutrition*, 235–263.

McLaren, L., & Hawe, P. (2005) Ecological perspectives in health research. *Journal of Epidemiology and Community Health* 59, 6–14.

Meier, P.P., Engstrom, J.L., Fleming, B.A., Streeter, P.L., & Lawrence, P.B. (1996) Estimating milk intake of hospitalized preterm infants who breastfeed. *Journal of Human Lactation* 12, 21–26.

National Board of Health and Welfare (2014) *Breast-feeding and Smoking Habits among Parents of Infants Born in 2012*. Stockholm: Centre for Epidemiology.

Organisation for Economic Co-operation and Development. (2011). Divided we stand: why inequality keeps rising. Country note: Sweden. http://www.oecd.org/sweden/49564868.pdf.

Parsons, H.M. (1974) What happened at Hawthorne?: New evidence suggests the Hawthorne effect resulted from operant reinforcement contingencies. *Science* 183, 922–932.

Reyna, B.A., Pickler, R.H., & Thompson, A. (2006) A descriptive study of mothers' experiences feeding their preterm infants after discharge. *Advances in Neonatal Care* 6, 333–340.

Scheff, T.J. (1997) *Emotions, the Social Bond, and Human Reality: Part/Whole*. Cambridge: Cambridge University Press.

Serenius, F., Sjors, G., Blennow, M., Fellman, V., Holmstrom, G., Marsal, K. et al. (2014) EXPRESS study shows significant regional differences in 1-year outcome of extremely preterm infants in Sweden. *Acta Paediatrica* 103, 27–37.

Spradley, J. (1980) *Participant Observation*. London: Cengage Learning.

Swedish Social Insurance Agency. (2012). Social Insurance Report, 2012:9 Stockholm: Swedish Social Insurance Agency.

van der Geest, S., & Finkler, K. (2004) Hospital ethnography: introduction. *Social Science & Medicine* 59, 1995–2001.

Vandenberg, K.A. (2007) Individualized developmental care for high risk newborns in the NICU: a practice guideline. *Early Human Development* 83, 433–442.

Wallin, L. (2009) Knowledge translation and implementation research in nursing. *International Journal of Nursing Studies* 46, 576–587.

Wierzbicka, A. (2009) Language and metalanguage: key issues in emotion research. *Emotion Review* 1, 3–14.

Wild, D., Grove, A., Martin, M., Eremenco, S., McElroy, S., Verjee-Lorenz, A. et al. (2005) Principles of good practice for the translation and cultural adaptation process for patient-reported outcomes (PRO) measures: report of the ISPOR Task Force for Translation and Cultural Adaptation. *Value Health* 8, 94–104.

World Health Organization. (2006). Bridging the 'Know–Do' Gap. Meeting on Knowledge Translation in Global Health 10–12 October 2005. Geneva, Switzerland: WHO.

Wrede, S., Benoit, C., Bourgeault, I.L., van Teijlingen, E.R., Sandall, J., & De Vries, R.G. (2006) Decentred comparative research: context sensitive analysis of maternal health care. *Social Science & Medicine* 63, 2986–2997.

7

NIGHT-TIME ON A POSTNATAL WARD

Experiences of mothers, infants, and staff

Catherine E. Taylor, Kristin P. Tully, and Helen L. Ball

Introduction

This chapter takes an experiential and emic approach to understanding night-time postnatal care in a UK hospital. We combine data from semi-structured interviews with descriptive video case studies to explore the experiences of mothers and their newborns, together with those of the postnatal ward staff. We interpret maternal and infant experiences and needs as biosocial processes. Cultural influences underlie the expectations, experiences, and interpretations of care on a postnatal ward at night. Research employing an experiential emic-focused approach can help to identify obstacles to optimal care for the mother–infant dyad and improve patient and staff experience of the hospital environment (Kleinman et al., 1978).

At the outset of this work, we were interested in understanding the barriers to breastfeeding on the postnatal ward (Ball et al., 2006). Previous research had identified maternal–infant separation as a key factor in the early supplementation of infants with human milk substitutes (e.g. formula, water) (Moore et al., 2012). In order to explore factors influencing breastfeeding outcomes, we conducted three related randomised controlled trials (RCT) that tested the effects of the postnatal ward proximity of new mothers and their infants for particular participant groups: 1) un-medicated vaginal births, 2) scheduled caesarean section births, 3) all term births. All of the participants in these studies expressed a prenatal intention to initiate breastfeeding. As part of these trials, we quantified maternal–infant interactions and infant feeding outcomes according to randomised infant sleep location: standard rooming-in with a stand-alone bassinet adjacent to the maternal bed, a side-car bassinet that locked onto the frame of the maternal bed and bedsharing. Observations were conducted overnight under infra-red light. The two bassinet types are shown in Figure 7.1.

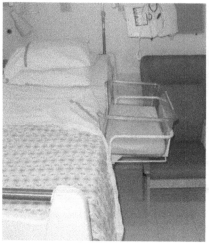 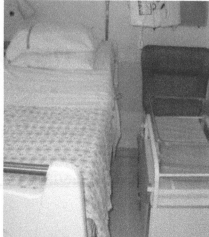

Side-car bassinet   Stand-alone bassinet

FIGURE 7.1 Bassinet types

Primary outcome data from the three original trials are published in Ball et al. (2006, 2011) and Tully and Ball (2012). Participants were asked to evaluate their night-time postnatal ward experiences during follow-up semi-structured interviews. For this chapter, qualitative reports were triangulated with descriptive case studies extracted from the video footage captured as part of these trials, building upon a method previously implemented by Volpe et al. (2013).

Background

While maternal and infant sleep behaviour and night-time infant care have been extensively studied in home and laboratory settings (Baddock et al., 2006, 2007; Ball et al. 2006; McKenna et al., 1997; Teti & Crosby, 2012; Volpe et al., 2013), the night-time and sleep-related experiences of mothers and newborn infants during their postnatal hospital stay has received only limited research attention. This is, however, an important issue; in 1989 the World Health Organization and UNICEF introduced the Baby-Friendly Initiative (BFI), including "10 Steps" for childbirth settings in support of promoting successful breastfeeding (WHO, 1989). Despite the fact that Step 7 recommends that mother and baby remain together day and night during the hospital stay, in many clinical locations mother and baby are still separated at night (Kurth et al., 2010). Night-time rooming-in (the practice of keeping infants in the same room as their mothers) is common practice throughout Europe (Moore et al., 2012) and becoming increasingly prevalent in the US, as hospitals there seek Baby-Friendly accreditation (Holmes et al., 2013). Rooming-in is associated with an increased prevalence of breastfeeding at hospital discharge in comparison with postnatal unit nursery care (Moore et al., 2012; Murray et al., 2007; Yamauchi and Yamanouchi, 1990).

However, Svensson et al. (2005) found that negative staff attitudes toward night rooming-in implicitly suggested to mothers that physical closeness with their baby during this period was not important. Furthermore, mothers who reported preference for infant nursery-care expressed more concern about their sleep and that of their babies while in hospital. Such concerns may be misplaced: a study examining the impact of rooming-in on maternal and infant sleep reported no difference in maternal sleep duration or quality between rooming-in or nursery care (Keefe, 1988), while infants experienced more quiet sleep, less crying, and more contact during rooming-in than during night-time nursery-care (Keefe, 1987). The benefits to mothers and infants of rooming-in, therefore, include facilitating successful breastfeeding initiation, enhanced bonding, and, for the infant, obtaining both comfort and sleep. However, for mothers, rooming-in can also present difficulties. An implicit expectation of rooming-in is that mothers or their family member/s will perform all infant care-giving activities, particularly at night when minimal staff assistance is available. Yet, family member presence may be restricted by hospital protocol. Additionally, maternal–infant interactions may be hindered by maternal pain, discomfort, and fatigue – particularly following childbirth with medical interventions such as episiotomies or operative delivery. The studies discussed here examined sleeping arrangements within the postnatal ward rooming-in environment. The purpose was to document the experiences associated with the key intention of rooming-in: mothers and newborns together to facilitate exclusive breastfeeding (Ball et al., 2006, 2011; Tully and Ball, 2012).

Theoretical approach

This chapter presents data gathered via a combination of methods chosen to elicit the emic and experiential perspectives of women (both patients and staff) inhabiting a UK tertiary hospital postnatal ward at night. An emic approach (sometimes referred to as "insider", "inductive", or "bottom-up") takes as its starting point the perspectives and words of research participants. In taking an emic approach, a researcher tries to put aside prior theories and assumptions in order to let the participants and data "speak" to them and to allow themes, patterns, and concepts to emerge (Lett, 1990). This approach is at the core of the Grounded Theory method, and is often used when researching topics that have not yet been heavily theorised. Some of its strength lies in its appreciation of the particularity of the context being studied, in its respect for local viewpoints, and its potential to uncover unexpected findings.

In contrast, an etic approach (sometimes referred to as "outsider", "deductive", or "top-down") uses as its starting point theories, hypothesis, perspectives, and concepts from outside the setting being studied. A researcher who takes an existing theory or conceptual framework and conducts research to see if it applies to a new setting or population is taking an etic approach (Lett, 1990). One of the strengths of the etic approach is that it allows for comparison across contexts and populations, and the development of more general cross-cultural concepts (Morris et al., 1999).

Drawing upon emic experiential perspectives is a central component of anthropological enquiry. We accomplish this here by combining observations of night-time events captured via video with maternal and staff experiences reported during interviews. Although this is not "video ethnography" in its proper sense, as we did not include discussion of events observed in the videos with the participants, the integration of the video and interview data provides a unique and useful approach for illuminating and understanding the night-time experiences of the mothers and staff of a UK postnatal ward – a setting where indirect observation via video triangulated by participant accounts is more feasible and acceptable than direct participant observation.

Research methodology: combining qualitative and observational data

Currently on UK postnatal wards, night-time is a period when visitors (including fathers) are normally prohibited, the frequency of patient–staff interactions is reduced, and mother–infant interactions are hidden from view by darkness and by curtains drawn around the beds. Consequently, in combining interviewing methods with naturalistic video observation, we had insight into experiences that would typically be out of sight to both the staff present on the hospital ward and researchers.

Participant responses about night-time infant care are also limited by memory, so video recording on the postnatal ward enabled an objective view of mother–infant behaviour with which to corroborate recalled experiences. Additionally, the observational data provided a more general insight into previously unacknowledged maternal–infant interactions during night-time postpartum hospitalisation. Observational data captured individually unique as well as common actions – important because behaviour is "not a static thing to be discovered" (Banks, 2001: 112). Health-related behaviours are increasingly conceptualised as a network of connections (Panter-Brick and Fuentes, 2008) and "while the overall pattern may be predictable, the interacting elements and process that produce [an] outcome are not" (Downe and McCourt, 2004: 14).

Qualitative data

Anthropological investigations are traditionally characterised by participant-observation. However, in the context of healthcare settings, the opportunity to have an extended presence can be restricted and problematic (Wind, 2008). Participation would mean becoming part of what is taking place – but when the researcher does not fit into the category of "visitor", "nurse/doctor", or "patient", the level of active engagement in events and activities within the hospital is limited. As it is therefore not possible to directly experience the night-time postnatal ward interactions as a researcher, we considered semi-structured interviews in conjunction with video footage to be a feasible and valuable alternative to traditional ethnography.

The relaxed format of the semi-structured interview method enables the researcher freedom to seek both clarification and elaboration on participant responses. This approach also provides a forum for the pursuit of topics that may not have originally been considered by the researcher as important, but may develop into significant themes within the findings (Bryman, 2008), and where the researcher has limited opportunities to interview someone (Bernard, 2002). In this series of studies interviews permitted insight into the perinatal experiences important to mothers. Carolan and colleagues (2006) asserts that these data are particularly useful for advancing "woman-centred" care by assisting midwives and other health professionals to subsequently provide more meaningful support.

Observational data

In the original studies upon which this chapter is based, the video data were analysed ethologically via quantitative coding of the frequency and duration of discrete behavioural categories defined according to an exhaustive and mutually exclusive catalogue of behaviours (behavioural taxonomy or ethogram) in order to permit statistical comparisons between groups (Martin and Bateson, 1993). However, in the present chapter we examine a selection of the videos as case studies, analysing them descriptively and in combination with maternal reports. The video case-study technique was used by Volpe et al. (2013) to understand the nature of rare experiences captured serendipitously during observational studies, borrowing the concept from learning studies (e.g. Goldman et al., 2007). Here we use video to illustrate and reinforce experiences described by participants, and reveal information about which midwives, researchers, and even (in some instances) mothers would be unaware.

The research studies

Our data are drawn from three distinct but related research studies consecutively conducted on the same UK tertiary-hospital postnatal ward between 2002 and 2010. Ethical and institutional approvals were obtained from Durham University and the local NHS Research Ethics Committees. All three projects involved prenatal enrolment of women pregnant with singletons and randomisation of the infant sleep location for postpartum rooming-in. At the study hospital, continuous rooming-in with a stand-alone bassinet was standard practice for all healthy dyads. All three studies examined the effects of mother–infant sleep proximity on the feeding and sleeping outcomes of mother–infant dyads. All were RCTs where dyads were randomised to different bassinet conditions during continuous rooming-in. Random allocation was employed to ensure that the factors that might affect maternal–infant interaction, known and unknown, would be evenly distributed across the trial groups.

Study details

Study 1 comprised an RCT of stand-alone bassinet, side-car bassinet, or bedsharing following un-medicated vaginal birth (Ball et al., 2006); study 2 comprised an RCT of side-car and stand-alone bassinet conditions following caesarean section childbirth (Tully and Ball, 2012), and study 3 comprised an RCT of side-car and stand-alone bassinet conditions for all mothers with healthy term births (Ball et al., 2011). Recruitment was conducted during pregnancy at prenatal clinics and classes. Enrolment for all three studies entailed the return of completed consent forms prior to childbirth and assignment of a study number. Exclusion criteria across the studies included premature delivery (< 37 gestational weeks) and intensive infant care. A research team member, who was not involved in recruitment, used a random-number table (studies 1 and 2) or a web-based randomisation service (study 3) to allocate participants to their groups. The first study, Ball et al. (2006), involved 64 mothers who gave birth vaginally to healthy term infants. These dyads were allocated to the stand-alone bassinet, a side-car bassinet, or bedsharing with the mother, using a bedrail. Intervention group participants (side-car or bedsharing) could revert to using the standard arrangement (stand-alone bassinet) on request.

The second study, Tully and Ball (2012), involved 35 term infants and their mothers who underwent scheduled, non-labour caesarean section childbirth. These participants were allocated to receive either the stand-alone bassinet or the side-car bassinet. The final study that we include here, Ball et al. (2011), was a large trial of 1200 participants where childbirth mode was not an inclusion or exclusion criterion and the participants were allocated to receive either the stand-alone bassinet or the side-car.

In the first two studies, a researcher conducted a semi-structured interview with the mothers and then set up a small camcorder and long-play videocassette recorder in the mother's postnatal room. The camcorder, which had "night-shot" capability that permitted filming in complete darkness, was mounted on a monopod clamped to the foot of the maternal bed and connected to a videocassette recorder that was housed in an attaché case positioned under the bed. Participants used a remote control to start recording once they were ready to settle for sleep and were requested to let the equipment record continuously for the duration of the 8-hour tape. Mothers and their midwives could stop the recording at any point. Participants were encouraged to care for their infants as usual and disregard the camera. Daytime behaviour was not filmed because of the variable presence of visitors and their interactions with the mother–infant dyad. Hospital policy excluded visitors (including the infant's father) overnight.

As part of the third study, a sub-sample of 64 participants were interviewed in person or by telephone at approximately six months postpartum. Interviews with 19 postnatal staff from the participating postnatal ward were also conducted (Taylor, 2013). For the staff interviews, a purposive sampling strategy was employed to ensure that participants represented a range of employment grades. These face-to-face interviews were conducted in a private room within the hospital once all of the mother–infant participants from study 3 had been discharged from the postnatal ward. A small gratuity was offered to the participants of all three studies in the form of gift cards.

Analyses

Interview responses were transcribed and thematically analysed by hand using a matrix format (study 1 and 2) or NVivo 8 software (study 3). The authors identified themes through an iterative process of grouping and regrouping the data. For this chapter, themes pertaining to night-time experiences of mothers and infants were selected; the themes presented below were also captured by observational video data. The latter had been ethologically coded using a behavioural taxonomy created in the Noldus Observer software package to categorise behavioural states and events. For the purposes of this chapter we reviewed the coded video data to find examples of behaviours or/experiences reported by participants during their interviews. The relevant video footage was then reviewed in real-time and a descriptive narrative account of the observation produced following the method implemented by Volpe et al. (2013).

Results

Five themes regarding night-time postnatal ward experiences were identified where qualitative and observational data substantially corroborated one another (see Table 7.1). These themes are presented below.

Theme 1 – Maternal need for support

Mothers' inability to independently access their infants while rooming-in at night was a prominent issue. Lack of assistance led women whose newborns were located in a stand-alone bassinet to make negative comments regarding this type

TABLE 7.1   Night-time postnatal ward experiences

Experiences described and observed
Maternal need for support
Response to infant cues
Negative experiences
Bedsharing as a way of coping
Insufficient staffing

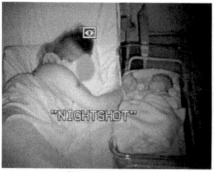 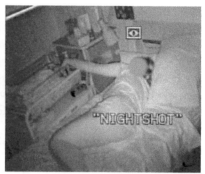

Side-car bassinet   Stand-alone bassinet

FIGURE 7.2 Mothers using stand-alone bassinets had difficulty reaching their infants

of rooming-in arrangement. Struggling to cope with infant needs through the night, while not feeling like a "nuisance" to midwifery staff, was a considerable problem to women. The mothers expressed reluctance to use their call-buzzer for staff assistance and they reported disappointment that the structure of the stand-alone bassinet impeded access to their infants (see Figure 7.2).

The challenge was particularly evident following caesarean section deliveries, after spinal or epidural anaesthesia during delivery, or among the mothers who were experiencing other pain or soreness. All women disliked the substantial manoeuvring they had to do to reach their newborns from the "awkward" and "clumsy" stand-alone bassinets. The corresponding maternal pain from these interactions was described as feeling as though they might "rip open". The mothers' "agony" was evidenced in videos by slow maternal movements and grimaces in the darkness. Further, many participants (not assigned to bedsharing) reported keeping their babies in the bed to avoid the need to repeatedly request help. Some women were particularly unhappy that their partners were not allowed to stay overnight:

> When he [husband] had to leave I would just start to cry…it was absolutely horrendous. I was totally alone, isolated.

In contrast, participants who received a side-car bassinet (or in study 1, a bedrail to facilitate bedsharing safety) expressed positive and enthusiastic responses about the usefulness of these rooming-in arrangements. The main advantage of the side-cars was described as facilitating access to infants without the need for assistance from staff. Staff also spontaneously commented that they perceived a reduction in "buzzing for assistance" when mothers were using side-car bassinets.

In one video of a mother–newborn dyad with a stand-alone bassinet, the woman sees her infant in the bassinet, leans forward, and winces as she slowly moves herself. It takes her several minutes to get up out of bed to stand next to the newborn. Then, after picking her infant up, the mother grimaces again when sitting back in bed and leaning back with her baby. Another mother described a similar experience:

> You can't get out of bed after a caesarean section. [with the stand-alone bassinet] You are leaning over and pulling on the [incision] wound. I feel upset because you can't move as quickly [after caesarean section] when the baby is crying. It is more of a struggle in the night. I have to ask others to change the nappy in night and as a new mother, you want to do that yourself.

The inability to fully care for infants while rooming-in with a stand-alone bassinet was repeatedly highlighted by mothers' hesitation to summon midwives for what could be considered straightforward tasks, such as placing an infant in a bassinet next to the bedside or changing the baby. One mother described the issue of infant access in relation to frequent night-time breastfeeding:

> When she was crying I had to ask somebody if she was OK and to help me because I had a completely numb leg and I couldn't move, so I think it would had been much more difficult for feeding and things through the night…so if every time I'd have wanted to feed her if I'd have had to ring for somebody, I think that would have made it much more difficult…I was really pleased I got the side-car bassinet and I think it was very beneficial in terms of encouraging breastfeeding and I think if I'd have felt less positive about it [breastfeeding] then I'd have been put off having to ask for help every time.

The majority of women who used the side-car bassinets on the postnatal ward offered that side-car bassinets should be the standard provision for postnatal ward care. Both mothers who were assigned the side-car bassinet and those who were allocated the stand-alone bassinet said that the side-car makes a considerable, positive difference to mothers' postnatal ward experiences. Maternal stress at the, sometimes overwhelming, tasks involved in infant and self care was also evident. Some mothers were observed crying in their beds while alone in the night. Women strongly emphasised the advantages of the close physical contact enabled by the side-car bassinets.

Theme 2 – Response to infant cues

Postnatal ward rooming-in arrangements impacted upon both mothers' responses to their infants' cues and the ability of the infants to bring their needs to their mothers' attention. As discussed above, many mothers with mobility issues after childbirth struggled with gaining access to their newborn. Time delays in responding to infants meant that the babies were often crying by the time their mothers had them in their arms. Mothers with the side-car bassinets (and in the first study those allocated to bedsharing) said that close physical contact with their infants enabled quick responses and frequent feedings. The visual and physical connection also served to reassure mothers that the baby was safe and well. During the daytime women who experienced rooming-in with stand-alone bassinets described keeping their babies in their arms, or a partner/family member holding the infant. These mothers would also have the baby in bed with them while they (women) were awake. However, through the night, when mothers using the stand-alone bassinets slept, this setup disrupted the dyads' connectedness.

From the infants' perspectives, the stand-alone bassinet created the need to expend more effort to attract their mothers' attention. This escalation of infant cues sometimes led to sustained crying, which in turn contributed to the level of noise on the ward that mothers complained about. Lack of maternal awareness of night-time infant cues is highlighted in the following sequence:

> At 2:35am a mother is sleeping and her baby, located in a stand-alone bassinet beside the mother's bed, begins to stir. Over the course of the next 10 minutes, the baby fully wakes and displays several rooting cues that signify he is ready to feed and searching for the mother's breast. Lying in a supine position, dressed in body-suit and socks with no blanket covering him, he spends several minutes squirming and rocking his head from side to side, kicking his feet, opening and closing his mouth, clicking his tongue, and mouthing his fists. He makes small snuffling and squeaking noises but does not cry. Meanwhile mother is asleep, in a supine position with a sheet pulled up to waist-height. Mother and baby are separated by a distance of no more than 30cm (1 foot), with the transparent plastic wall of the stand-alone bassinet between them – yet the mother is oblivious to her baby's waking, readiness to feed, and his attempts to locate her. As they are on separate surfaces, she cannot feel him move and the infant cannot reach her (see Figure 7.3).

In the above example, a feeding opportunity is missed when the baby gradually stops rooting and returns to sleep. The mother slept throughout this period without stirring.

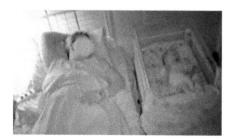

FIGURE 7.3 Mother sleeps through feeding cues

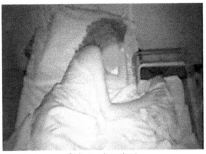
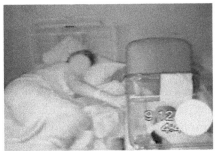

Side-car bassinet   Stand-alone bassinet

FIGURE 7.4   Mothers with stand-alone bassinets had difficulty soothing infants

When mothers were aware of their infants' need to be removed from the stand-alone bassinet, some described frustration at not being able to respond effectively. Multiple mothers were observed lying on their sides in bed and reaching out to rock or jiggle the bassinet frame (see Figure 7.4). These attempts to soothe their newborns while waiting for midwifery assistance were usually ineffective, as one video description illustrated:

> The baby is crying in the stand-alone bassinet. The mother has her hand over edge of the bassinet to reach her baby, but can only touch him with her fingertips. She presses the call-buzzer for the midwife, and shakes the frame of the bassinet in an attempt to comfort the baby while remaining lateral in her bed, waiting for a midwife to attend. Baby continues crying.

In contrast, mothers with the side-car bassinets responded to their babies quickly by patting and stroking them (see Figure 7.4). This possibility for side-car participants of having infants within reach was described as "just tremendous". In various videos with side-car bassinet participants, mothers placed, and often slept with, a hand on their newborns' chests. One such mother reported the ease of touching and reassuring her baby. Another mother compared her study experience with the side-car with her previous experience with a stand-alone bassinet:

> Actually the side-car is really good. I can be a lot more responsive quicker. I pick him up [out of the side-car] straight away whereas it takes me a good few minutes to get up out of bed. My little girl [previous baby] had been left crying [on the postnatal ward with the stand-alone bassinet]. I found this a lot easier. It was ideal when he was asleep. I could put my hand on him when he niggled.

In summary, when women's movements were constrained after their deliveries, the stand-alone bassinet was viewed by the mothers as a direct impediment to their infant caretaking. The postnatal ward rooming-in arrangements provoked dramatically different types of interactions with their infants. These differences contributed to maternal concerns about infants suffering from impaired maternal access, breastfeeding difficulties, and worry whether infants could breathe when they coughed or displayed other concerning behaviour. Some mothers were also anxious that their babies would disturb other dyads on the ward if they cried, and so they were tasked not only with the responsibility of newborn care, but also with "keeping the peace" during the night.

Theme 3 – Negative experiences

A small proportion of women participating in the studies had infants taken out of their rooms for a period during the night. The explicit purpose of most of these separations was to enable the mother to get more sleep, without the "burden" of breastfeeding what one midwife described as "greedy" infants, or the interruption of other caretaking behaviours. The idea of non-continuous rooming-in was introduced by staff on multiple occasions. Although some women described welcoming the opportunity for time apart from their babies and one mother (allocated a stand-alone bassinet) said that she requested the midwives take her baby for part of the night, another mother attributed the actions by the midwifery staff as contributing to her early cessation of breastfeeding.

> I feel really quite cross now when I look back on it 'cos I was trying to breastfeed…they came in and said all the other babies are going to be taken away so that you and the other women on the ward can get some sleep and that made me feel sort of pressured…they took him away and I found out actually afterwards that they gave him a bottle [on two consecutive nights] and they didn't tell me about it. It sounds ridiculous 'cos I'm not a woman who cries but I just started to weep…that to me really undermined what I was trying to do.

Another mother, whose baby would not settle in the stand-alone bassinet, had concerns that her baby's crying was going to disturb others on the ward but was also worried that she would roll on her infant if she fell asleep with him next to her in bed. She described asking a member of staff for formula milk at night-time as way of settling her infant in the stand-alone bassinet, something she said she might not have done if her infant was beside her in the side-car arrangement. This was a common theme in study 3 with the majority of "top-up" formula feeds (used by a third of mothers on the postnatal ward) occurring at night-time; mothers described these "top-ups" as attempts to stop their baby from crying and to induce infant sleep.

No participants or their infants were observed, or otherwise documented, as having experienced harm. However, situations that put babies at risk arose

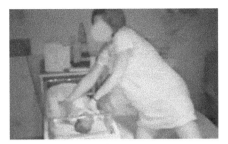

FIGURE 7.5   Mother has to stand on her knees to retrieve infant

in relation to the interaction of the stand-alone cot structure with limited maternal mobility. Those mothers who were mobile often stood on their knees to reach their infant (see Figure 7.5). The distance and height of the stand-alone bassinet led some mothers to provide poor support to their infants when moving them compared with the access enabled by the side-car. Infants were viewed with suboptimal neck support, being shuffled in a stand-alone that tipped sideways under the weight of a mother's arms as she was leaning on it to retrieve him from her position in bed, and an infant being dropped several inches into a stand-alone bassinet adjacent to the mother's bed (see Figure 7.6). The participant who accidentally dropped her baby into the stand-alone bassinet could not maintain contact with her infant from her position sitting on the bed. After the baby was in the bassinet, she got up onto her knees, scooted over to him, and verbally apologised.

Theme 4 – Bedsharing as a way of coping

The isolation felt by mothers on the night-time postnatal ward, and the inconvenience of the stand-alone bassinets led to many women bedsharing with their babies for sleep. The main reasons given for this arrangement were for feeding or to settle a fractious infant and some of these mothers reported falling

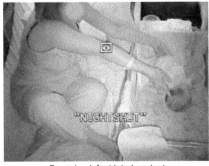

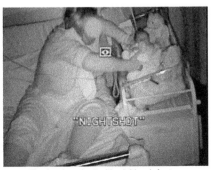

Dropping infant into bassinet   Tipping bassinet with picking infant up

FIGURE 7.6   Mothers with limited mobility had difficulty moving babies

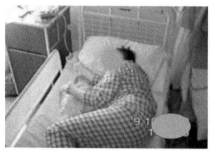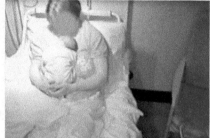

FIGURE 7.7 Mothers fell asleep with babies in more or less safe ways

asleep; one commented she found it was getting "a bit silly" frequently getting in and out of bed:

> It [side-car bassinet] certainly would have made being able to hold Adam easier and even helped me to get a little bit of rest. To have him so close to me, 'cos sometimes when a baby cries they just want a bit of contact, to know that you're there, so just being able to put your hand in and touch him, that's all they want. Whereas with the other ones [stand-alone bassinet] even having them up next to the bed, 'cos of the cupboard thing that they are on…there's still a good half foot between you…and they're quite high up as well, they're not the most practical of things.

Women stated that when they removed their infant from the bassinet to join them in the bed their intention was to stay awake. However, we observed several mothers who fell asleep with their babies in their arms instead of returning them to the bassinet. Unintended bedsharing introduced potential risks to the infants. A problem with this scenario, especially when the mother was in a reclining position, was the risk of the baby sliding off her chest to the floor when the mothers' arms relaxed (see Figure 7.7). In study 1 when mothers were randomised to bedshare with a bedrail they slept alongside their babies, often feeding in a side-lying position and the bedrail prevented the possibility of falls.

In another video, a post-caesarean section mother can be seen breastfeeding her infant in bed, and then watching the infant sleep on a pillow on her lap for a few minutes. The woman then looks at the stand-alone bassinet adjacent to her bed, and then back at her infant multiple times. She seemed to be debating about whether it was "worth" the effort to move her infant. In the end the participant fell asleep with the infant still on the pillow on her lap.

Theme 5 – Insufficient staffing

Many women commented that care on the postnatal ward was compromised by staff being too busy to offer sufficient support, particularly with breastfeeding.

Furthermore, accounts provided by multiparous mothers indicated staff often assumed such women did not require support leaving them feeling "forgotten about":

> I couldn't get her to feed at all in the hospital...I didn't actually feed her until I got home...she [midwife] came and more or less just said "here's these nipple shields they might help" and they didn't...I felt really stressed by the fact that I hadn't fed her...I felt really pressured to breastfeed on the ward but not given any help to do it... they were just really, really busy.

> I had to wait a while for someone to come 'cos they were always really busy you know, so I'm that kind of person who doesn't like to bother people you know so I just waited to catch somebody and it was sorta later on in the day and someone came, and I'd been trying myself before then, and I said I just can't get him to latch on...and she did help me to get it started and I did manage to feed him but then after that I couldn't get him to do it again.

In a hectic environment, some women felt that their needs were not significant in relation to the staff's overall work. Furthermore, assistance that was delivered in a rushed manner was described as little benefit to helping women gain knowledge and confidence in infant care. Consequently, in the absence of sufficient support during the daytime, the women were even less able to cope with issues that arose during the night-time period when staffing levels and presence on the postnatal ward was further reduced.

Delay in postnatal ward staff support of mothers at night-time can undermine breastfeeding. In one night-time filming session, a health assistant (technician) asked how the mother was doing as she took her blood pressure. After the mother mentioned breastfeeding difficulty, the technician did not respond or seek midwifery assistance. The upset woman was left on her own. The participant later buzzed for a midwife and asked to be brought a bottle of formula, to which the midwife offered breastfeeding support. However, the woman gave her infant the formula. In another example, maternal discomfort and tiredness after ceasarean section childbirth was exacerbated by a delay in painkiller provision by the midwives. During the observation period, a participant asked a midwife for the pharmaceuticals and although the midwife said she would oblige, she did not return for 50 minutes. By then, the woman was sleeping and was woken by the midwife's return.

Insufficient staffing levels was not only a problem discussed by the mothers; all of the staff interviewed identified this to be the main constraint of care they delivered. Several staff mentioned that the side-car bassinet alleviated some of the demands on their time in addition to providing mothers with greater satisfaction of being able to independently meet their infants' needs.

> I think a lot of mams kind of give up on breastfeeding if they have to keep buzzing us, especially as they can see it's busy on here [the ward] and they don't have somebody, a port of call for help, especially when it's busy and we're short staffed.

When discussing postnatal breastfeeding support, the overwhelming consensus amongst the staff was that although breastfeeding was high on the agenda for importance, the reality of what the staff were able to deliver was frustratingly inadequate both in quality and quantity. This was attributed to low staffing levels, high workload expectations and rapid patient turnover. Overall, the staff felt this problem was beyond their control. Lack of comprehensive breastfeeding support created feelings of anxiety and guilt amongst some members of staff when their attention was needed elsewhere: "It's whoever's needs are most, you just have to decide 'cos you can't tear yourself in half."

The following account offers a valuable insight into the high-pressured environment in which staff are typically working. It is notable that the description of the workload appears to be dominated by medical procedures and checks without mention of time being allocated to practical and emotional support for mothers who require help when providing care for their infant:

> For next door's 24-bedded ward [surgical ward] there's three midwives on and we're full today, so that's eight to nine women each and they're all newly sectioned so they've all had major surgery, they need all the medical, you know, drips, catheters, wound dressing, observations, blood pressures done, so you have all that and we have all the transitional care babies, so all tube feeding and that sort of thing so if you have eight of those or nine of those then you're pretty full on, I mean you have 18 people really for one midwife really 'cos it's mums and babies, this is a 24-bedded ward here [non-surgical ward] and there are two midwives on this morning.

Discussion

By identifying five themes regarding night-time interactions in the postnatal ward, we have sought to draw attention to the experiences of mother–infant dyads as well as the perspectives of the staff involved in their care. Emerging from all three of our studies was evidence that "traditional" rooming-in, with infants in stand-alone bassinets adjacent to maternal hospital beds, was unsatisfactory. Alternate models for rooming-in using either bedsharing or side-car bassinet arrangements were both reported by mothers, and observed, to improve the postnatal ward experiences of women, their infants, and hospital staff.

A key concern of mothers in our studies was their ability to respond to their infant's needs. Mothers who bedshared or had the side-car bassinets were less reliant on hospital staff and reported that their overall postnatal ward experiences were greatly enhanced by unhindered access to their newborns. The stand-alone bassinet was found to be both a physical and emotional barrier between mother and baby. This arrangement contributed to infant crying (which has also been referred to as the "separation distress call", Christensson et al., 1995), delays in breastfeeding and, in many instances, maternal distress and pain when attempting to access the baby.

In situations where mothers struggled to independently care for their newborns, or infants were distressed, staff sometimes offered formula and/or removal of infants from the mothers' rooms in attempts to facilitate maternal sleep. Similarly, Heinig (2010) showed that staff attitudes regarding formula supplementation to combat "problem" infant crying and maternal fatigue were difficult to change. Further, Furber and Thomson's (2006) study revealed that midwives reported to have knowingly engaged in "breaking the rules" regarding their hospital's breastfeeding policy by giving formula milk to infants at night on a regular basis. This was a practice that the midwives involved regarded as responsible care rather than deviant behaviour, yet they chose to hide their actions from both the mothers and their peers due to concerns over how their intervention would be received. As with Heinig's (2010) research, staff explained their behaviour as benefiting mothers who were experiencing fatigue or difficulties following childbirth. In some instances, the midwives justified their actions by suggesting that it was essential to maintain breastfeeding motivation in some mothers. This claim is in direct contrast to the findings by McAndrew et al. (2012) that receipt of additional feeds (formula, water or glucose) on the postnatal ward was associated with an increased likelihood of stopping breastfeeding in the early weeks after delivery. Furthermore, Declercq et al.'s (2009) research revealed that hospital practices conflicting with BFI guidelines (notably formula/water supplementation) were more likely to result in unfulfilled intentions to exclusively breastfeed at one week, particularly in first-time mothers.

Various studies have documented that separation of newborns from their mothers not only undermines breastfeeding but impacts also upon on the physical and emotional well-being of both mother and baby (Bergman et al., 2004; Morgan et al., 2011; Winberg, 2005). Night-time separation and/or formula being given to infants without the mother's permission or maternal report of pressure to consent to otherwise not medically "necessary" formula feeds have been documented in multiple other studies (such as Beeken and Waterston, 1992; Raisler, 2000; Whelan and Lupton, 1998). Such "culture-lag" in the biomedical system is defined as the persistence of patterns of behaviour long after the clinical rationale for the practices has been dismissed (Kroeger, 2004). As Dykes (2006) points out, these interventions serve to restore culturally embedded, shared notions of "order" to the postnatal ward which is likely to underpin why such practices perpetuate or are not strongly challenged by mothers.

The video observations uncovered a number of previously unknown, or at least unacknowledged, safety issues with rooming-in on the postnatal ward, such as when mothers encountered difficulty manoeuvring infants in and out of the stand-alone bassinet or when infants were brought into bed as a means of coping with night-time infant care. In-hospital infant drops and falls to the floor are dramatic yet under-researched events; one study that examined data from 18 hospitals in the US over a three-year period reported 14 infant falls (Monson et al., 2008). The circumstances surrounding the falls were documented as follows: four falls occurred in the delivery room, two in the hallway when a nurse was wheeling a bassinet, one when an infant was placed in an infant swing, and seven when a parent fell asleep whilst holding the infant in a hospital bed (or in one instance a reclining chair). Notably, six of the seven falls from a parent's arms occurred between 1:30am and 9:00am. In another study, Helsley et al. (2010) gathered data from seven US hospitals over a two-year period and reported nine cases of newborn falls. The incidents were reported as follows: one fall occurred in the context of a father falling asleep holding an infant in a chair, one when the mother tripped on her intravenous line when getting out of bed holding the infant, two when the mother was repositioning or transferring the infant to a stand-alone bassinet whilst remaining in the bed, one when the mother fell asleep when breastfeeding (not specified if this was in the bed or in a chair), and four occurred when the mother fell asleep holding the infant in bed. In all but two cases the event occurred during the night or in the early hours of the morning and the parent and not a member of staff initially discovered all fallen infants. Helsley et al. conclude that greater attention to newborn safety is required in the engineering of hospital equipment. They argue that the distance between the bed and the stand-alone bassinet discourages the mother from using it and suggest that a side-car bassinet arrangement could reduce the number of in-hospital infant falls. Observational methods, therefore, are a useful tool to divulge contextualised accounts of the physically or emotionally harmful situations that mothers and infants may encounter on the postnatal ward at night-time. These interactions are otherwise invisible to both staff and researchers employing traditional ethnographic methods.

The emic descriptions we amassed of the postnatal ward from both mothers and staff reinforce Dykes' (2006) analysis of an occasionally rushed, chaotic, and fragmented approach to medical care. Dykes (2006) reports that mothers complained that staff rarely "touched base" with them except to carry out routine checks. This left some women feeling that summoning a member of staff for breastfeeding or infant care support was an unwarranted diversion from more important or urgent tasks. Dykes discusses how the unpredictability of events on the postnatal ward means that staff may be moved at any time to treat another patient, leading to a working philosophy to "get the job done" in case the situation suddenly changed. Consequently, relationships between mothers and midwives are suboptimal and staff often feel stressed. Overall, the postnatal ward faces considerable obstacles to the implementation of change (Bilson and Dykes, 2009; Cox, 2009; Dykes, 2006; Dykes and Flacking, 2010; Edwards et al., 2011; Hughes et al., 2002; Kirkham, 1999; Schmied et al., 2011). The damaging effect of this environment on mothers is reflected in studies linking a negative postnatal ward experience with unfulfilled breastfeeding intentions (Burns et al., 2010; Nelson, 2006; Renfrew et al., 2012; Tarkka et al., 1998; Thomson and Dykes, 2011) and postnatal depressive symptoms (Astbury et al., 2010; Huang and Mathers, 2008; Kitzinger, 2012). In contrast, individualised, sensitive lactation support increases maternal confidence and satisfaction of postnatal care in hospital (Bäckström et al., 2010). Further, a systematic review by Renfrew et al. (2012) recommended a proactive approach to breastfeeding support. The report concluded that support within community and hospital settings, that is only offered reactively to women who seek out help, is likely to be ineffective at increasing any or exclusive breastfeeding duration.

A novel issue to emerge from our analyses involves the cultural expectations and environmental ecology of UK hospitals at night and their impact on postnatal care. Night-time staffing levels and service provision (such as absence of management staff, visitors, catering etc.) strongly signal that night-time is considered "down-time" in these settings. Implicit here is the assumption that fewer midwives are needed on the ward overnight compared with daytime because mothers and newborns are expected to be primarily sleeping at night, with mothers in their beds and infants in their stand-alone bassinets. Assumptions are of a quiet environment, lack of disturbance, few demands, and no problems that require urgent or specialist attention. Well-meaning staff understandings are that mothers need to sleep. In this mindset, if infants need attention, then an appropriate role of the staff is to give the mothers "a break". This care may include feeding the baby formula without maternal consent or knowledge and/ or removing the newborn from the mothers' rooms. The cascade of maternal–infant separation events unwittingly harms at least lactation physiology, if not other aspects of bidirectional maternal–infant processes such as attachment.

Such institutional expectations and staff assumptions as discussed above fail to incorporate either local hospital ecology or maternal–newborn biology. Multiple studies have reported that UK hospitals are poorly designed to promote "down-time", rest, or sleep among patients. Sleeping with strangers in communal wards, unfamiliar and uncomfortable beds, lack of light screening between areas, the noises of patients and staff, constant bright lighting of hallways and corridors, all serve to impede sleep (Armstrong et al., 2004; Meltzer et al., 2012; Southwell and Wistow, 1995; Topf and Davis, 1993). Expectation of prolonged bouts of both maternal and newborn sleep is also inconsistent with the short sleep and feeding cycles of infants, and the need for mothers to nurse frequently in the early post-partum period in order to increase prolactin production and facilitate lactogenesis II, the production of mature breast milk.

Our research suggests a more appropriate conceptualisation of postnatal ward dynamics that involves: 1) extensive and dynamic night-time activity, 2) many new mothers being at least sore and at worst immobile and therefore requiring physical assistance and emotional support, 3) newborn "expectation" to maintain physical contact with their mothers after childbirth and infant protest when they feel separated from their caregivers, 4) infants and mothers, unless under the influence of labour analgesia or experiencing medical complications, feeding frequently throughout the night and often benefiting from assistance or support, and 5) hospital furniture and ward arrangements either constraining or promoting particular ward interactions. Overall, the combination of descriptive and ethnographic approaches allowed us to gain emic insight into the mother–baby experience of night-time on the postnatal ward. The findings can be translated into clinical changes to facilitate responsiveness to infant cues and maternal self-care.

Strengths and limitations of approach

The extended, naturalistic recordings of mother–infant and maternal–staff interactions obtained through overnight filming captured contextualised data that were otherwise inaccessible. Combining objective coding of behavioural recordings with qualitative data analyses offers a holistic understanding of the processes that contribute to health outcomes. An additional strength of our research approach is that including images and video clips (with explicit consent from participants) alongside summary statistics and participant quotes in scientific and policy presentations can be an effective way convey the study findings.

Drawbacks to observational research include the extensive time and financial investment required for continuous coding of such extended observations. Our studies were limited by the use of single, standard-definition cameras that recorded at fixed angle and zoom. Some behaviours could have been missed due to lack of recording clarity or when participants moved out of range. Ongoing parent–infant sleep studies use multiple, high-definition infrared cameras that permit wide-angle recording and zooming-in on particular areas of interest during the coding process. A further constraint of observational research is that some people are averse to being videoed. The self-selective nature of volunteering for research means that the behaviours of participants may systematically vary from those who do not take part. Also, some clinical staff expressed concern to our research team that information from the study observations might be used to "reprimand" them. Therefore, the interactions recorded for the research projects may have differed from standard care.

Conclusions

The research approach introduced in this chapter enables us to have unique insight into ways to make postnatal wards more family friendly. The use of side-car bassinets, having lactation support available and expected through the night, and facilitating partners to stay overnight are a few of the many protocol changes that are consistent with the 10 Steps to Successful Breastfeeding (WHO, 1989) and can be further tested to extend this standard level of evidence-based care. Future research may benefit from featuring parental (maternal and paternal) satisfaction, depressive symptoms, and anxiety as outcome measures alongside infant feeding outcomes. In our studies reported here, although most women were unhappy with their postnatal ward care, none of them formally complained or reported serious errors. This suggests that without research that utilises the combination of extended filming and participant questioning to understand the observed behaviours, experiences such as the difficulties that many new mothers experience with the stand-alone bassinets while rooming-in on the postnatal ward, may never be brought to light officially. The stand-alone bassinet may not just be inconvenient for mothers, it may be an unnecessary breastfeeding obstacle and an institutionalised risk for infants.

References

Armstrong, D., Kane, M., Reid, D., McBurney, M. & Aubrey-Rees, R. 2004. *The Role of Hospital Design in the Recruitment, Retention and Performance of NHS Nurses in England.* London: Commission for Architecture and the Built Environment (CABE). Available at: http://webarchive.nationalarchives.gov.uk/20110118095356/http:/www.cabe.org.uk/files/the-role-of-hospital-design-appendices.pdf

Astbury, J., Brown, S., Lumley, J. & Small, R. 2010. 'Birth events, birth experiences and social differences in postnatal depression.' *Australian Journal of Public Health,* 18(2):176–184.

Bäckström, C., Wahn, E. & Ekström, A. 2010. 'Two sides of breastfeeding support: experiences of women and midwives.' *International Breastfeeding Journal,* 5(1):20.

Baddock, S.A., Galland, B.C., Bolton, D.P., Williams, S.M. & Taylor, B.J. 2006. 'Differences in infant and parent behaviors during routine bed sharing compared with cot sleeping in the home setting.' *Pediatrics,* 117(5):1599–1607.

Baddock, S.A., Galland, B.C., Taylor, B.J. & Bolton, D.P. 2007. 'Sleep arrangements and behavior of bed-sharing families in the home setting.' *Pediatrics,* 119(1):e200–207.

Ball, H.L., Ward-Platt, M.P., Heslop, E., Leech, S.J. & Brown, K.A. 2006. 'Randomised trial of infant sleep location on the postnatal ward.' *Archives of Disease in Childhood,* 91:1005–1010.

Ball, H.L., Ward-Platt, M.P., Howel, D. & Russell, C. 2011. 'Randomised trial of sidecar crib use on breastfeeding duration (NECOT).' *Archives of Disease in Childhood,* 96:360–364.

Banks, M. 2001. *Visual Methods in Social Research,* London: Sage Publications.

Beeken, S. & Waterston, T. 1992. 'Health service support of breast feeding – are we practising what we preach?' *British Medical Journal,* 305(6848):285–287.

Bergman, N., Linley, L. & Fawcus, S. 2004. 'Randomised controlled trial of skin-to-skin contact from birth versus conventional incubator for physiological stabilization in 1200- to 2199-gram newborns.' *Acta Paediatrics,* 93:779–785.

Bernard, H.R., 2002. *Research Methods in Anthropology: Qualitative and Quantitative Methods,* Lanham, MD: AltaMira.

Bilson, A. & Dykes, F., 2009. 'A biocultural basis for protecting, promoting and supporting breastfeeding.' In Dykes, F. & Hall Moran, V. (eds). *Infant and Young Child Feeding: Challenges to Implementing a Global Strategy,* Oxford: Wiley-Blackwell.

Bryman, A. 2008. *Social Research Methods,* Oxford: Oxford University Press.

Burns, E., Schmied, V., Sheehan, A. & Fenwick, J. 2010. 'A meta-ethnographic synthesis of women's experience of breastfeeding.' *Maternal and Child Nutrition,* 6:201–209.

Carolan, M., Andrews, G.J. & Hodnett, E. 2006. 'Writing place: a comparison of nursing research and health geography.' *Nursing Inquiry*, 13(3):203–219.

Christensson, K., Cabera, T., Christensson, E., Uvnäs-Moberg, K. & Winberg, J. 1995. 'Separation distress call in the human neonate in the absence of maternal body contact.' *Acta Paediatrics*, 84:468–473.

Cox, S. 2009. 'Altering hospital maternity culture current evidence for the ten steps to successful breastfeeding.' *Medications and More Monthly Newsletter*, 13(11).

Declercq, E., Labbok, M.H., Sakala, C. & O'Hara, M. 2009. 'Hospital practices and women's likelihood of fulfilling their intention to exclusively breastfeed.' *American Journal of Public Health*, 99(5):929–935.

Downe, S. & McCourt, C. 2004. 'From being to constructing: reconstructing childbirth knowledge.' In Downe, S. (ed.). *Normal Childbirth Evidence and Debate*. Edinburgh: Churchill Livingstone.

Dykes, F. 2006. *Breastfeeding in Hospital: Mothers, Midwives and the Production Line*, London and New York: Routledge.

Dykes, F. & Flacking, R. 2010. 'Encouraging breastfeeding: a relational perspective.' *Early Human Development*, 86:733–736.

Edwards, N., Murphy-Lawless, J., Kirkham, M. & Davies, S. 2011. 'Attacks on midwives, attacks on women's choices.' *Aims Journal*, 23(3) http://www.aims.org.uk/Journal/Vol23No3/attacks.htm

Furber, C.M. & Thomson, A.M. 2006. 'Breaking the rules in baby-feeding practice in the UK: deviance and good practice?' *Midwifery*, 22(4):365–376.

Goldman, R., Pea, R., Barron, B. & Derry, S.J. (eds). 2007. *Video Research in the Learning Sciences*, London: Routledge.

Heinig, M.J. 2010. 'Addressing maternal fatigue: a challenge to in-hospital breastfeeding promotion.' *Journal of Human Lactation*, 26(3):231–232.

Helsley, L., McDonald, J.V. & Stewart, V.T. 2010. 'Adressing in-hospital "falls" of newborn infants.' *The Joint Commission Journal on Quality and Patient Safety*, 36(7):327–333.

Holmes, A.V., McLeod, A.Y., & Bunik, M. 2013. 'ABM Clinical Protocol #5: peripartum breastfeeding management for the healthy mother and infant at term, revision 2013.' *Breastfeeding Medicine: The Official Journal of the Academy of Breastfeeding Medicine*, 8(6):469–473.

Huang, Y. & Mathers, N. 2008. 'Postnatal depression – biological or cultural? A comparative study of postnatal women in the UK and Taiwan.' *Journal of Advanced Nursing*, 33(3):279–287.

Hughes, D., Deery, R. & Lovatt, A. 2002. 'A critical ethnographic approach to facilitating cultural shift in midwifery.' *Midwifery*, 18(1):43–52.

Keefe, M.R. 1987. 'Comparison of neonatal night-time sleep–wake patterns in nursery versus rooming-in environments.' *Nursing Research*, 36(3):140–144.

Keefe, M.R. 1988. 'The impact of infant rooming-in on maternal sleep at night.' *Journal of Obstetric, Gynaecologic, & Neonatal Nursing*, 17:122–126.

Kirkham, M. 1999. 'The culture of midwifery in the National Health Service in England.' *Journal of Advanced Nursing*, 30(3):732–739.

Kitzinger, S. 2012. 'Rediscovering the social model of childbirth.' *Birth*, 39(4):301–304.

Kleinman, A., Eisenberg, L. & Good, B. 1978. 'Culture, illness, and care: clinical lessons from anthropologic and cross-cultural research'. *Annals of Internal Medicine*, 88:251–258.

Kroeger, M. 2004. *Impact of Birthing Practices on Breastfeeding: Protecting the Mother and Baby Continuum*, Sudbury, MA: Jones and Bartlett.

Kurth, E., Spichiger, E., Zemp Stutz, E., Biedermann, J., Hösli, I. & Kennedy, H.P. 2010. 'Crying babies, tired mothers – challenges of the postnatal hospital stay: an interpretive phenomenological study.' *BMC Pregnancy Childbirth*, 10:21.

Lett, J. 1990. 'Emics and etics: notes on the epistemology of anthropology.' In Headland, T.N., Pike K.L. & Harris, M. (eds). *Emics and Etics: The Insider/Outsider Debate*. Frontiers of anthropology, v. 7. Newbury Park, CA: Sage Publications. 9:127–142.

Martin, P. & Bateson, P.P.G. 1993. *Measuring Behaviour: An Introductory Guide*, Cambridge: Cambridge University Press.

McAndrew, F., Thompson, J., Fellows, L., Large, A., Speed, M. & Renfrew, M.J. 2012. *Infant Feeding Survey 2010: Summary*. Department of Health. http://www.hscic.gov.uk/catalogue/PUB08694/Infant-Feeding-Survey-2010-Consolidated-Report.pdf

McKenna, J.J., Mosko, S.S. & Richard, C.A. 1997. 'Bedsharing promotes breastfeeding.' *Pediatrics*, 100(2 Pt 1):214–219.

Meltzer, L.J., Finn Davis, K. & Mindell, J.A. 2012. 'Patient and parent sleep in a children's hospital.' *Pediatric Nursing*, 38(2):64–71.

Monson, S.A., Henry, E., Lambert, D.K., Schmutz, N. & Christensen, R.D. 2008. 'In-hospital falls of newborn infants: data from a multi-hospital health care system'. *Pediatrics*, 122;e277–e280.

Moore, E.R., Anderson, G.C., Bergman, N. & Dowswell, T. 2012. 'Early skin-to-skin contact for mother and their healthy newborn infants (Review)'. *The Cochrane Library*. http://www.cochrane.org/CD003519/PREG_early-skin-to-skin-contact-for-mothers-and-their-healthy-newborn-infants

Morgan, B.E., Horn, A.R. & Bergman, N.J. 2011. 'Should neonates sleep alone?' *Biological Psychiatry*, 70:817–825.

Morris, M.W., Leung, K., Ames, D. & Lickel, B. 1999. 'Views from inside and outside: integrating emic and etic insights about culture and justice judgment.' *Academy of Management Review*, 24(4):781–796.

Murray, E.K., Ricketts, S. & Dellaport, J. 2007. 'Hospital practices that increase breastfeeding duration: results from a population-based study.' *Birth,* 34(3):202–211.

Nelson, A.M. 2006. 'A metasynthesis of qualitative breastfeeding studies.' *Journal of Midwifery & Women's Health,* 51:e13–e20.

Panter-Brick, C. & Fuentes, A. 2008. 'Health, risk and adversity: a contextual view from anthropology.' In Panter-Brick, C. & Fuentes, A. (eds). *Health, Risk and Adversity*, New York: Berghahn, 2:1–10.

Raisler, J. 2000. 'Breastfeeding experiences of low income mothers.' *Journal of Midwifery & Women's Health,* 45(3):253–263.

Renfrew, M.J., McCormick, F.M., Wade, A., Quinn, B. & Dowswell, T. 2012. 'Support for health breastfeeding mothers with health term babies (Review).' *The Cochrane Library*. http://onlinelibrary.wiley.com/doi/10.1002/14651858.CD001141.pub4/abstract

Schmied, V., Gribble, K., Sheehan, A., Taylor, C. & Dykes, F. 2011. 'Ten steps or climbing a mountain: a study of Australian health professionals' perceptions of implementing the baby friendly health initiative to protect, promote and support breastfeeding.' *BMC Health Services Research*, 11(1):208.

Southwell, M.T. & Wistow, G. 1995. 'Sleep in hospitals at night: are patients' needs being met?' *Journal of Advanced Nursing*, 21:1101–1109.

Svensson, K., Mattiesen, A.S. & Widström, A.M. 2005. 'Night rooming-in: who decides? An example of staff influence on mother's attitude.' *Birth,* 32(2):99–106.

Tarkka, M.-T., Paunonen, M. & Laippala, P. 1998. 'What contributes to breastfeeding success after childbirth in a maternity ward in Finland?' *Birth*, 25(3):175–181.

Taylor, C.E. 2013. *Post-natal Care and Breastfeeding Experiences: A Qualitative Investigation Following a Randomised Trial of Side-Car Crib Use (NECOT Trial)*. PhD Thesis: Durham University. Available at: http://etheses.dur.ac.uk/10530/1/Taylor_Thesis_Final.pdf

Teti, D.M. & Crosby, B. 2012. 'Maternal depressive symptoms, dysfunctional cognitions, and infant night waking: the role of maternal night-time behavior.' *Child Development*, 83(3):939–953.

Thomson, G. & Dykes, F. 2011. 'Women's sense of coherence related to their infant feeding experiences.' *Maternal and Child Nutrition*, 7(2):160–174.

Topf, M. & Davis, J.E. 1993. 'Critical care unit noise and rapid eye movement (REM) sleep.' *Heart & Lung*, 22(3):252–258.

Tully, K.P. & Ball, H.L. 2012. 'Postnatal unit bassinet types when rooming-in after cesarean birth: implications for breastfeeding and infant safety.' *Journal of Human Lactation*, 28(495).

Volpe, L.E., Ball, H.L. & McKenna, J.J. 2013. 'Nighttime parenting strategies and sleep-related risks to infants.' *Social Science and Medicine*, 79:92–100.

Whelan, A. & Lupton, P. 1998. 'Promoting successful breastfeeding among women with a low income.' *Midwifery*, 14:94–100.

WHO. 1989. A joint WHO/UNICEF Statement 'Protecting, Promoting and Supporting Breastfeeding: The Special Role of Maternity Services.' Geneva: World Health Organization. Available at: http://whqlibdoc.who.int/publications/ 9241561300.pdf

Winberg, J. 2005. 'Mother and newborn baby: mutual regulation of physiology and behaviour – a selective review.' *Developmental Psychobiology*, 47:217–229.

Wind, G. 2008. 'Negotiated interactive observation: doing fieldwork in hospital settings.' *Anthropology & Medicine*, 15(2):79–89.

Yamauchi, Y. & Yamanouchi, I. 1990. 'The relationship between rooming-in/not rooming-in and breast-feeding variables.' *Acta Paediatrica Scand*, 79(11):1017–1022.

8

FATHERS' EMOTIONAL EXPERIENCES IN A NEONATAL UNIT

The effects of familiarity on ethnographic field work

Kevin Hugill

Introduction

In this chapter I draw upon an auto/biographically informed ethnographic doctorial study into the early emotional experiences of fathers in a neonatal unit to reflect on some of the realities and practicalities of conducting ethnography in a field which the researcher is both familiar with and known in. In considering some of the key challenges and complexities of undertaking ethnographic fieldwork in a familiar field I explore the effects of this familiarity upon how respondents and researcher relationships interacted as new research-oriented relationships struggled to take precedence.

Encountering parenthood in a neonatal unit is an unplanned for and novel situation for most parents. Parents of preterm infants seem to have a different experience compared with those with healthy term infants. Reviews of neonatal parenthood studies worldwide consistently highlight the relationship between preterm birth and increased and enduring levels of parental stress and the long-lasting effects these experiences can have (Cleveland 2008; Treyvaud 2014). However, much of the research has used mothers as key informants to the relative omission of fathers' perspectives. This situation has left a void in our understanding of how both parents experience preterm birth and having their infant admitted to a neonatal unit. This relative lack of description from fathers of preterm infants and how these experiences affect them was the starting point for my doctoral study. I report in more detail on the findings from this study in Hugill and Harvey (2012), Hugill et al. (2013) and Hugill (2014).

In order to understand the design choices, conduct and findings of any study it is important to establish its setting. The following section sets out some of the contextual background of my study. Firstly I briefly describe my place in the study with respect to aspects of my personal and professional biography. Secondly to aid readers unfamiliar with the health speciality of neonatal care, a brief description of how hospital-based neonatal care is organised in the UK and the study site is provided. After establishing this background I then go on in the following section to discuss why I chose ethnography for my study method. After this I describe some of the methodological imperatives that informed my approach and briefly describe the study's theoretical framework or 'lens' through which the analysis of primary data was structured and interpreted. The later section and subsections of this chapter concern the conduct of ethnography in a familiar health care setting before finally offering some concluding thoughts.

The contexts of this study

My place in the study

Early on in my study I was working (in a nursing capacity) for the National Health Service (NHS) Trust that managed the neonatal unit (the study site). Towards the end of data collection I moved away and was employed in a different organisation. In the past I had worked on the neonatal unit in a variety of nursing capacities for around thirteen years in total, but at the time of the study I no longer worked there. When I began my employment in the study site neonatal unit I was the only male nurse working in the department. In later years other men were employed as nurses in the department. However, overall they remained a very small minority with never more than four people out of complement of over ninety nurses. In addition I am a father of preterm children (now grown). Consequently because of this past association I retained some of the attributes of an 'insider'. More accurately my identity could be better described as that of a 'quasi-insider-outsider' in that I retained insider knowledge but I was no longer a formal part of the setting.

Neonatal care in the UK and the study site

The work of neonatal units is characterised by technology-driven health care with a focus on saving the lives of ever-lower gestational age infants. For some this generates tensions between ensuring the correct balance between human centredness and technological ability is upheld. The environments are physically closed and widely considered to have a unique organisational subculture (Wilson et al. 2005). Ethical dilemmas around the margins of viability for life, the effects of high-tempo working, cot occupancy and capacity to admit feature regularly in discussions about neonatal services.

Most infants born in the UK are healthy and require little in the way of medical attention; however, some through prematurity or illness require admission to a neonatal unit. Admission rates to neonatal units vary geographically and this is mainly linked to the incidence of preterm birth and indices of socio-economic deprivation (Weightman et al. 2012). In broad terms around 8–13 per cent of newborn babies spend time in a neonatal unit (Goldenberg et al. 2008). Most of these infants spend only a short time under medical care; however, approximately 1–3 per cent of all births require intensive care resources. These infants are the sickest and generally the most preterm and can spend many months in hospital before they are able to go home to live with their parents.

In the UK, hospital-based neonatal care is provided under the NHS funded through direct taxation. Following a national review in 2003 (DH 2003) neonatal care was reorganised along lines that categorised individual units by the intensity of medical and nursing care available. Essentially this meant that level 1 neonatal units provided the most basic level of care, with level 2 providing some more complex care and level 3 units the most intensive medical and nursing care. Despite some recent modifications and further local and national healthcare reorganisation this categorisation remains broadly adhered to.

The site of my study was designated as a level 3 unit and was situated in a large NHS teaching hospital which provided services to a population of around 320,000 people. At the time the unit admitted around 500 infants per year and had eleven intensive/high dependency and additional special care category cots. Intensive/high dependency was in an open plan room and special care (low dependency) cots were in two rooms nearby.

Why ethnography?

Ethnography has acquired almost as many meanings and practices as it has researchers using it as a research methodology and method. This lack of coherence can be problematic in understanding ethnographic research accounts. According to Ellis and Bochner (2000) ethnographies, despite their varying method and methodological assertions, only differ in the degree of emphasis they place upon the self, culture and the research process. The nature of ethnography as method and methodology offers the promise of combining and integrating different philosophical and design ideas. Whilst there is no singular consensual definition of its nature, it does have a number of trademark features. These include a naturalistic focus on cultural interpretations of complex social phenomena, the use of multiple data sources and the need to establish a balance between emic and etic (insider and outsider) perspectives (Hammersley and Atkinson 2007). Fathers' experiences, like many social phenomena, are multidimensional and viewing any such complex phenomena from a single perspective may weaken our understanding. Based on my study's purpose and desire to reveal multiple perspectives on fathers' experiences, an ethnographic approach was deemed most appropriate. Ethnography, it was felt, held the promise of revealing previously unacknowledged facets of fathers' experience during this time.

Participant observation is one of the hallmarks of ethnography but it is not the only source of data. Direct observational data is frequently supplemented by interviews both informal and more arranged; however, in deciding upon which sources of data to use a key question is one of relevance to the research aim. In research settings where respondents and researcher potentially might know each other, managing issues of trust, disclosure and confidentiality requires thoughtful consideration at the design stage and throughout (McDermid et al. 2014). In my study, seeking to strike a balance between emic and etic perspectives, I set out to use non-participant observation, informal interviews with respondents and some more in-depth interviews with some fathers. Carrying out in-depth interviews with health professionals was rejected as potentially problematic given my past acquaintances. To counter any potential problems and create some distance I chose to opt for an alternative ethnographic data collection tool. Preliminary thematic networking analysis (Braun and Clarke 2006) of observation and interview data was used to construct a qualitative ethnographic survey for administration to health professionals. Schensul and LeCompte (2013) define this approach thus: 'An ethnographic survey is based on concepts and scales that emerge from or are adapted to the culture of the study site' (p. 243).

Using site-specific structured approaches can offer a way to turn ethnographic data into quantitative instruments or test their relationships (Schensul and LeCompte 2013). In essence, because the ethnographic survey I used was developed from observational and interview data collected at the study, I sought to do the latter. One motivation was to test out preliminary analytic understandings of the data. There were other motivations behind this particular choice of approach to collecting data which included:

- A desire to capture a broader range of perspectives from health professionals not involved in data collection so far
- To invite a larger number of respondents to participate than observation alone could include
- To meet timeliness deadlines for data collection.

Schensul and LeCompte (2013) suggest that ethnographic surveys are carried out face-to-face with respondents, though they accept that this might not always be possible and that self-administered surveying is an acceptable alternative. In this study, because I was previously known to some respondents, the survey provided them with a means to take part anonymously.

Informing methodological imperatives and analytic lens

Ethnography largely dispels the idea that the researcher can be a dispassionate individual on the outside looking in. Despite claims to the contrary research is never carried out in total isolation; all studies are situated within a cultural framework of pre-existing knowledge, understandings, values and beliefs. Ethnographic data collection, by its very nature, involves establishing relationships with respondents and living with them though their experiences.

Consequently ethnographers operate as more than just a tool of data collection and the 'personhood' of the researcher becomes an integral part of the ethnographic account.

In social inquiry curiosity about research topics often derives from direct experience and observation of the world, tacit theories and political commitments (Mills 1959). Denzin and Lincoln (1998: xviii) develop this point and suggest 'many researchers study problems anchored in their personal biographies'. However, 'It is inaccurate to assume that *all* [original italics] research is grounded in the autobiographies of researchers' (Letherby et al. 2013: 2–3). Nevertheless insight into the researcher's self can help in understanding how the research was conceived, conducted and interpreted. I am in broad agreement with Stanley and Wise (1993), in that: 'it isn't possible to do research (or life) in such a way that we can separate ourselves from experiencing what we experience as people (and researchers)' (Stanley and Wise 1993: 159–160).

The auto/biographical research method, though not exclusive to feminist research, is nevertheless rooted in feminist ideas about the joint endeavour and interconnectedness between researcher and respondent when researching women's lives (Letherby 2003). Davies (1999) concluded that some acknowledgment of auto/biographical perspectives is essential in situations where the researcher is a member of the group under study to ensure research and researcher transparency. Auto/biographical informed writing and research, whilst now widely accepted, was in the past criticised as being mainly about the researcher's self and consequently dismissed as self-indulgent and narcissistic; but this misses the point. Mykhalovskiy (1996) suggests that this critique is based upon an erroneous premise: that research work exists in which the researcher's auto/biography does not feature at some level. For example, anecdotally many nurses undertaking research for a higher degree study topics anchored in their everyday practice experience, i.e. their professional biography. Nevertheless few would declare their topic choice to be inherently affected by their personal biography. I recall that at the start of my study I was similarly reticent in this respect despite having worked in neonatal care for many years and also being a father of four prematurely born children (all now adult). However, early conversations with my supervisory team introduced me to ideas about how our personal and professional biographies interact; this was an important step towards the hybrid auto/biographical ethnographic approach adopted in my thesis. In sum: 'auto/biographical method isn't about self-reference for the sake of it' (Hugill 2012: 31). Instead this method can, through reflexivity, set out and make transparent additional components of the research process (such as the interpretive lens / world view of the researcher). This transparency can add to credibility claims, help to counter the insularity of many research accounts and furthermore reveal some of the hidden or silent spaces of doing research (ethnography).

Emotion work

Emotions are a part of everyday life and one of the main components of interpersonal interaction. Nevertheless people's emotions and emotional states are not always easy to know even when people are closely familiar with each other. Invariably we interpret others' emotions through our own frame of reference and past experience, and this can be problematic. Studies of how people manage their emotions in everyday and extreme situations increasingly feature in the literature. Emotion work is a sociological concept that has become widely used to structure the study of a person's control of emotional expression, particularly within organisational and work environments. Hochschild (1979; 2003) conceptualised the effort individuals exert to manage their own and the emotions of others as 'emotion work'. This concept belongs to a group of theoretical ideas about emotion labelled 'dramaturgical theories of emotions' (Turner 2009). This phrase acknowledges the work of Goffman (1959) and his influence on Hochschild's thinking. Goffman (1959) argued that society could be explained through the metaphor of a theatrical play in which people sought to present themselves to an audience. Hochschild (1979) argued that the experience and management of emotions are dictated by culturally determined rules (normative, feeling and display rules) and that these are learnt through socialisation. Crucially these rules are not fixed; they can differ with age, gender, time, place and social context (Bolton 2005).

In summary, ideas expressed in the term emotion work are a response to the physical, psychosocial and cultural situations that impose demands on individuals to emotionally react in a particular way, whether or not they truly feel that way. Few studies have explored men's emotion work in family life and work and little is known about men's emotional management in relation to neonatal care and this was why the concept was chosen for my study.

Conducting ethnography in familiar health care settings

Gathering research data through fieldwork observation can pose complex, theoretical, ethical and practical difficulties. Issues around research design, developing rapport, obtaining consent, negotiating access, ethical dilemmas and managing data all feature. Despite this most books on ethnography poorly explain how familiarity affects these issues. In the remainder of this chapter I seek to partially redress this. The following subsections focus upon some of the practical issues (and solutions) from carrying out participant observations and gathering data. In particular I describe and reflect upon some of the features and tensions in respondent–researcher relationships met during this study and what measures were put in place and how my behaviour was modified in order to carry out data collection successfully. In particular, nurse and researcher role conflict, researcher presentation and respondent reactivity are explored.

Being a quasi-insider-outsider

Familiarity with a potential study site can have advantages. For example prior understanding of cultural nuances, tacit behaviour rules and knowledge about how the organisation works can help with negotiations with formal and informal gatekeepers in gaining access to 'backstage' areas. For ethnographers this is balanced by some notable drawbacks. For example gaining insight into tacit cultural aspects can be harder if the observer has complex emotional ties to respondents (McDermid et al. 2014; Steibel et al. 2014). Also it is quite common for researchers to have concerns that over-familiarity can risk undermining the integrity of the research in some way. Indeed many health professional researchers take considerable effort to ensure a dispassionate and uninvolved identity in their research. This strategy is met with varying amounts of success and to my mind might not be entirely desirable or unavoidable for those with dual professional and researcher responsibilities towards respondents.

Group membership is complex and cannot be easily defined (Simmons 2007; Evans et al. 2013). As my own experiences suggest group memberships, particularly in work settings, are not fixed and change over time and circumstance. Being a nurse doing research in health can have benefits. Leslie and McAllister (2002) argue that having a nursing identity in health research settings can help researchers gain privileged access to intimate and sensitive areas of respondents' lives. Furthermore, nurses' familiarity with talking about these sensitive and intimate topics can enable them to readily empathise and respond to respondent emotions. However, it is important to remember that the benefits of having a shared experience in developing rapport with and understanding respondents' lives is not confined to nurse researchers alone.

In contrast, having a pre-existing nursing identity can impede access to some study environments due to protocol and professional hierarchies (Pereira de Melo et al. 2014). Bell and Nutt (2002) state that in general insiders are exposed to additional problems, tensions and risks which can be both practical and ethical in nature. For nurse-researchers this can involve feeling additional moral responsibilities and difficulties in balancing research and organisational roles (Cudmore and Sondermeyer 2007; Houghton et al. 2010). Additionally it can create ambiguity over nursing and nurse-researcher identities causing role conflict and confusion (Simmons 2007; Ashton 2014). I concur with these assessments and the following reflective subsections: 'getting involved', 'wearing "my" clothes and wearing working clothes' and 'field note taking' highlight why this is the case.

Getting involved

Fieldwork is a social process and as such not always predictable and can be a source of threat to researchers. Reviewing published fieldwork accounts reveals considerable categorical range in actual and feared threats both in and from the field. These include fears about physical, emotional, moral and professional hazards (Blackman 2007; Howell 2007; Bloor et al. 2010; Houghton et al. 2010). The following incident involving the father of a dying infant occurred quite early on in my fieldwork and illustrates some of tensions inherent in being viewed as an insider by some respondents. On the day in question I knew that their infant was dying and to give the family some privacy I had moved away from the vicinity to an adjacent room. After a short time the father of the infant sought me out, he said:

> 'Can I have a word with you in private?' [Field note]

'Yes', I replied, not knowing what it was about but fearing some complaint about my research conduct. This was not the case. He went on to say that he remembered I had told him I was a nurse and explained that he would like me, as a man who was not a family member, to shave his child's head prior to a religious ceremony. After speaking with staff and gaining their approval I agreed to do this. I completed the task watched by family members. Afterwards the grandmother gave me £5; from previous experience I knew that declining the money would be disrespectful. The money was put into the unit's charitable funds. Later I was told that the infant had died. Afterwards I reflected upon this incident in my research diary:

> I have only done three observations; it seems I can't get beyond my neonatal nurse label. Today I got involved with a dying baby, at dad's request and stopped just observing. [Field note]

Despite my initial frustrations I had some time later after further reflection annotated this entry:

> In spite of this, I felt good about today, why? [Field note]

I knew that the infant's death was unavoidable and I felt that my actions helped to support and prepare the family for this inevitability. I realised this was a good thing to do that on a deeper level resonated with my personal experiences.

During this study to reinforce my researcher identity and down-play any expectations around my nursing identity I had set out to only carry out non-participatory observations, in part to avoid professional entanglements. However, my intentions in this respect were often frustrated. From early on in my research it quickly became clear that my professional identity compromised this plan. In reality the degree of participation in activities with respondents fluctuated and can be best viewed as sliding backwards and forwards on a pragmatic and philosophical continuum.

Wearing 'my' clothes and wearing working clothes

A consistent theme for ethnographers is the need to engage with the process of fieldworker presentation. Dress, speech, prior skills and other personal attributes like gender, age, and social status can affect respondent and researcher relations (Hammersley and Atkinson 2007). Typically ethnographers make use of three common approaches when presenting themselves to potential respondents, specifically as an academic researcher, as one of you or as a learner; each has merits.

In one ethnographic study Hunt, a midwife-researcher, recalled her choice of clothing: 'I chose to wear a skirt, blouse and white coat' (Hunt and Symonds 1995: 45). She went on to justify this choice and her wanting to distinguish her status as a researcher and not a midwife. Adding, it would be unusual unless a member of the public to not be wearing some sort of uniform in this area (a midwifery department) but dressing as a midwife might lead to expectation she was available to participate in clinical work. However, her choice of a white medical overcoat inadvertently had one other unanticipated effect: 'the white coat and its symbol of medical supremacy proved to be a passport to all areas' (Hunt and Symonds 1995: 45).

The traditional medical white coat is rarely worn by neonatal and paediatric clinicians and wearing one in a neonatal unit would mark the individual as an outsider. Previously, in my work, I had encountered similar situations whereby my choice of clothing affected my reception. During everyday work (a clinical nursing and managerial role), I wore either a nursing uniform (navy smock) or office-wear (shirt and tie) depending upon the day's activities. During fieldwork I consciously ensured that I never wore this type of clothing. In addition, I conducted myself differently by purposefully avoiding talk about organisational matters, instead focusing solely upon research matters. Despite this strategy, early on health care professionals seemed sometimes confused and sought clarification about my role, for example:

> 'Morning Kevin, are you a worker or a researcher?' [Field note]

This comment reveals something of an oxymoron for nurse researchers doing fieldwork in a familiar environment: that doing research fieldwork = doing nothing. It betrays a familiar stereotype in some areas of nursing: that you are only 'working' if you are engaging in providing patient care and all other activities are not real work.

On occasions nurses chose to purposefully ignore that I was there to do research and requested my assistance, for example during one period of observation when the unit had absent staff and a lot of infants were requiring feeding at the same time one nurse said:

> 'Kevin, I'm really sorry but can you give us a hand for a while with the feeds [nasogastric tube feeding]?' [Field note]

In order to maintain a positive respondent relationship I often felt under obligation to acquiesce to these requests; a strategy that Evans et al. (2013) suggest can help to alleviate anxieties about the research in nurse participants and ease the researcher's acceptance in the field. Sometimes my consent was not sought but seemingly implied merely by my presence and health professionals' knowledge about me. One example of this occurred during a period of observation in a lower infant dependency room; the nurse said to other staff present:

> 'I'm going to break now, Kevin's around in here if you need anything.' [Field note]

According to Coffey (1999) successful fieldwork is synonymous with proactive management of researcher image. In this study, my attempts at impression management (after Goffman 1959) went beyond my choice of clothing and included other elements such as demeanour and speech. In this, I was concerned with presenting a plausible researcher identity that was acceptable to respondents and yet remained compatible and credible with my other identities (personal, professional and organisational). In reality, my attempts to stage-manage how others saw me were not entirely successful. Being an ethnographer and doing ethnography is a negotiated state, as Madden insightfully observed, 'it's not always the choice of ethnographers themselves as to how they wish to be in the field' (Madden 2010: 81).

Field note taking

Naturalistic participant observations are often credited with gathering data with minimal impact upon those studied and accurately capturing how things are despite the research activity (Lincoln and Guba 1990). However, this view makes a number of contestable assumptions, including about how things are naturally and that respondents under observation behave naturally. Early explanations of the effects of an observer on activities were often referred to as 'Hawthorne effects' and were viewed by some as problematic interfering with the natural flow of events. However, the term (Hawthorne effect) is of questionable utility as it lacks precision, has multiple meanings and is often used to refer to any uncontrolled-for effect (Chiesa and Hobbs 2008). In addition, it negates the bidirectional flow of influence between research participant and researcher. Consequently I use the term 'respondent reactivity' as it better describes the bidirectional flow of these research and researcher effects and how observational researchers and respondents interpersonally interact.

Prior to starting participant observations I purchased a distinctive notebook unlike any other used in the site. This was again attempting to stage-manage my perception by others and convey that I was engaged in something different from anything they might have seen me do before. It quickly became apparent that taking field notes was affecting people's behaviours. Like others (see Madden 2010), I was not prepared for the extent to which my presence and my past would influence the tone of interactions with respondents. At the beginning of fieldwork I noted that health care professionals who were normally quite talkative became less so and others became focused and engaged in their tasks. One day a nurse remarked jovially as I entered the intensive care room:

'Kevin's got his book again so you better all be working.' [Field note]

This comment caused laughter amongst those present and whilst the comment was humorous there are a number of possible explanations. It could represent genuine humour in a situation where she felt secure. Alternatively, it could signify an attempt to redress a perceived power imbalance or inform others about my intentions. Whatever the reason, clearly, my attempts to make unobtrusive field notes were less successful than I had hoped.

After this episode I changed the way I recorded data. As Madden advises, in order to continue to gather data: 'be prepared to put down the pen and paper' (Madden 2010: 128). I no longer carried a notebook around and instead left it in another room where I could intermittently retire to write up key phrases, prompts and the like for later integration. Whilst this had the effect of making my note-taking less obtrusive I noticed that there was more inclination by nurses to engage me in clinical activities.

In order to mitigate any misconceptions about covert observation I adopted two behaviours to make it obvious that I was engaging in research observation, rather than anything else. After entering the unit, I would make an obvious show of placing my notebook in an adjacent room and perhaps more importantly, where possible, I would sit down. Sitting down in the clinical areas was something that health care professionals rarely did during the daytime, except when helping mothers or feeding infants. These seemingly simple details ensured that my recording of field notes remained overt, yet unobtrusive.

Monahan and Fisher (2010) highlight that concerns about respondent reactivity impacting on and corrupting the research feature frequently in criticisms of ethnography. However, using examples from their own research they concluded that fears about respondents self-censoring their behaviour are broadly unfounded. Findings from my own study (Hugill 2014) concerning how parents and health professionals make critical judgements about one another's behaviours and motives support this argument.

Being a nurse and nurse-ethnographer

According to Alvesson and Sköldberg (2009) researchers and respondents affect each other mutually and continually. Concern about the appropriateness of fieldworker behaviours are highlighted as a source of tension and debate across broad areas of ethnographic work (Blackman 2007). For nurse-researchers anxieties about clinical responsibilities towards respondents regularly feature in research accounts (see Hunt and Symonds 1995; Cudmore and Sondermeyer 2007). Indeed some nurse-researchers report that they temporarily abandoned their research and reverted to former clinical roles (Burden 1998).

One example that illustrates some of this disquiet is described by Hunt (Hunt and Symonds 1995) as she recalled observing a difficult birth which she did not intervene in, reflecting afterwards that she should have acted at the time. After this experience she concluded that health professionals have a moral and professional obligation to act when the need arises, regardless of any research context. Being a nurse I was aware that my conduct within the study site would be judged by research ethics and professional codes of conduct. As such, it was important that I sought to balance these expectations.

One way to incorporate and clarify research governance and clinical responsibilities is to prepare an ethical protocol beforehand. This protocol can be designed to address broad areas of nursing and research conduct, for example ensuring patient safety or treating life-threatening events (Houghton et al. 2010). In my early conversations with formal and informal gatekeepers (of the study site) just such a protocol was negotiated in order to plan for potential issues. The principles guiding this protocol were professional and research standards and codes of conduct. In addition it recognised the priority to safeguard the rights, welfare and interests of respondents above my research agenda. To support me it was agreed that I have an organisation-based supervisor whom I would regularly meet with weekly during fieldwork to debrief. Although at first inspection ethical protocols might seem uncontentious, this is not the case. They are open to interpretation, for example, in terms of beneficence is it the parents, infants (implies researcher is right) or professional colleagues (where intervention might unbalance self-esteem and learning) together with the nature of events (are we understanding them correctly without full knowledge of circumstances)?

Regardless of how they do it, nurse-researchers need to simultaneously balance the expectations of professional practice together with those of research governance. Walker (1997) suggested that nurse-researchers occupy neither the land of practice nor research; instead they criss-cross the narrow boundaries between the two, the 'borderlands'. It is the need to repeatedly negotiate traversing this border that is the source of anxiety. For me a more powerful metaphor is that nurse-researchers live in the 'debatable land', a much broader geography in which to dwell. The term 'debatable land' historically referred to the disputed area of the border between England and Scotland, particularly between the late 13th and 16th centuries (Fraser 1971; Moffat 2008). More recently the term has come to be used, as here, beyond its immediate geographical and political senses to draw attention to any area of contested or unresolved debate. Nurse-researchers inhabit a space where boundaries exist but they are imprecise, indeterminate and fluid, allowing the obligations of practice and research to interact and coexist simultaneously.

For me, Reinharz (1997) offers perhaps the best explanation of research reflexivity, describing it as critical self-reflection during which there is explicit consideration of the researcher, the research and its participants and findings. Transparently and reflexively accounting for the researcher in the research process can enhance credibility and claims of morally responsible research conduct (Alvesson and Sköldberg 2009). However, research settings that link with our own personal and professional biographies can pose potential for hazard in terms of emotional danger and exposure to professional criticism. In addition numerous commentators have suggested that prior acquaintance with research settings can put researchers in potentially vulnerable situations. For nurse-researchers this familiarity can also create professional dilemmas and concern over role, themes I have explored in this chapter. Respondents in my study engaged in a complex arrangement of relationships with me as a person, nurse and researcher. Questions about the nature and conduct of these relationships are integral to reflexive accounting. Reflexively setting out the interpretive lens, how the field affects the researcher and the researcher affects the field can make the research process more transparent. 'Our biography encroaches on our research and the ways in which we conduct it and should be accounted for in our research writing' (Hugill 2012: 32). Despite this, overtly reflexive research accounts, whilst common in research carried out by women, are with some exceptions (see Robertson 2006 for example) less evident in male researchers' writing; this chapter adds to this limited body of writing.

Concluding thoughts

The main aim of my study was to gain a variety of perspectives on the emotional management experiences of fathers of preterm infants. In addition the study has also generated insight into the nature and conduct of researcher and respondent relationships during ethnographic fieldwork. There is no doubt that ethnographic fieldwork is harder and more complex than it is often presented to novice researchers. It seems that there are many opportunities for researchers to become entangled in events which can pose risk to study and researcher integrity. The need to systematically account for the effects of these relationships is endorsed by my findings.

During data collection the clothes I wore affected how respondents viewed and sometimes utilised me. Tensions over the duality of nurse-researcher roles (role conflict), observer effects on respondents and the effects of fieldworker image management were evident. It seems that fieldwork shapes and constructs researcher identity in ways not entirely defined or predicted by researchers themselves. In my study respondents placed me within a social landscape that was defined by their previous experiences. Importantly the experiences related in this chapter have also had effects relating to a broader canvas of me as 'ethnographer', 'neonatal nurse' and 'man and father'. Nevertheless, the issues highlighted in this chapter have begun to account for and reveal aspects of the 'hidden ethnography' of fatherhood study and carrying out research in a neonatal unit.

References

Alvesson, M and Sköldberg, K (2009) *Reflexive Methodology: New Vistas for Qualitative Research*. 2nd edition. London: Sage.

Ashton, S (2014) Researcher or nurse? Difficulties of undertaking semi-structured interviews on sensitive topics. *Nurse Researcher* 22(1): 27–31.

Bell, L and Nutt, L (2002) Divided loyalties, divided expectations: research ethics, professional and occupational responsibilities. In: M Mauthner, M Birch, J Jessop and T Miller (Eds) *Ethics in Qualitative Research* (pp. 70–96). London: Sage.

Blackman, S (2007) 'Hidden ethnography': crossing emotional borders in qualitative accounts of young people's lives. *Sociology* 41(4): 699–716.

Bloor, M, Fincham, B and Sampson, H (2010) Unprepared for the worst: risks of harm for qualitative researchers. *Methodological Innovations Online* 5(1): 45–55. DOI: 10.4256/mio.2010.0009

Bolton, SC (2005) *Emotion Management in the Workplace*. Basingstoke: Palgrave Macmillan.

Braun, V and Clarke, V (2006) Using thematic analysis in psychology. *Qualitative Research in Psychology* 3(2): 77–101.

Burden, B (1998) Privacy or help? The use of curtain positioning strategies within the maternity ward environment as a means of achieving and maintaining privacy, or as a form of signalling to peers and professionals in an attempt to seek information or support. *Journal of Advanced Nursing* 27(1): 15–23.

Chiesa, M and Hobbs, S (2008) Making sense of social research: how useful is the Hawthorne effect? *European Journal of Social Psychology* 38(1): 57–74.

Cleveland, LM (2008) Parenting in the neonatal intensive care unit. *Journal of Obstetric, Gynecological and Neonatal Nursing* 37(6): 666–691.

Coffey, A (1999) *The Ethnographic Self: Fieldwork and the Representation of Identity*. London: Sage.

Cudmore, H and Sondermeyer, J (2007) Through the looking glass: being a critical ethnographic researcher in a familiar nursing context. *Nurse Researcher* 14(3): 25–35.

Davies, CA (1999) *Reflexive Ethnography: A Guide to Researching Selves and Others*. London: Routledge.

Denzin, NK and Lincoln, YS (Eds) (1998) *The Landscape of Qualitative Research: Theories and Issues*. Thousand Oaks, CA: Sage.

Department of Health (DH) (2003) *Report of the Neonatal Intensive Care Services Review Group*. London: Department of Health.

Ellis, C and Bochner, AP (2000) Autoethnography, personal narrative, reflexivity: researcher as subject. In: NK Denzin and YS Lincoln (Eds) *Handbook of Qualitative Research*. 2nd edition (pp. 733–768). London: Sage.

Evans, A, Pereira, D and Parker, J (2013) Categorising the nurse-researcher during fieldwork: 'one of us' or 'one of them'? *Journal of Research in Nursing* 18(8): 707–717.

Fraser, GM (1971) *The Steel Bonnets: The Story of the Anglo-Scottish Border Reivers*. London: Collins Harvill.

Goffman, E (1959) *The Presentation of Self in Everyday Life*. London: Penguin.

Goldenberg, RL, Culhane, JF, Iams, JD and Romero, R (2008) Preterm birth 1: epidemiology and cause of preterm birth. *The Lancet* 371(9606): 75–84.

Hammersley, M and Atkinson, P (2007) *Ethnography: Principles in Practice*. 3rd edition. London: Tavistock.

Hochschild, AR (1979) Emotion work, feeling rules, and social structure. *American Journal of Sociology* 85(3): 551–575.

Hochschild, AR (2003) *The Managed Heart: Commercialization of Human Feeling*. 20th anniversary edition. Berkeley, CA: University of California Press.

Houghton, CE, Casey, D, Shaw, D and Murphy, K (2010) Ethical challenges in qualitative research: examples from practice. *Nurse Researcher* 18(1): 15–25.

Howell, N (2007) Human hazards in fieldwork. In: ACGM Robben and JA Sluka (Eds) *Ethnographic Fieldwork: An Anthropological Reader* (pp. 234–244). Malden MA: Blackwell.

Hugill, K (2012) Auto/biographical method and its potential to contribute to nursing research. *Nurse Researcher* 20(2): 28–32.

Hugill, K (2014) Father–staff relationships in a neonatal unit: being judged and judging. *Infant* 10(4): 128–131.

Hugill, K and Harvey, M (2012) *Fatherhood in Midwifery and Neonatal Practice*. London: Quay.

Hugill, K, Letherby, G, Reid, T and Lavender, T (2013) Experiences of fathers shortly after the birth of their preterm infants. *Journal of Obstetric Gynecological and Neonatal Nursing* 42(6): 655–663.

Hunt, S and Symonds, A (1995) *The Social Meaning of Midwifery*. London: Macmillan.

Leslie, H and McAllister, M (2002) The benefits of being a nurse in critical social research practice. *Qualitative Health Research* 12(5): 700–712.

Letherby, G (2003) *Feminist Research in Theory and Practice*. Buckingham: Open University Press.

Letherby, G, Scott, J and Williams, M (2013) *Objectivity and Subjectivity in Social Research*. London: Sage.

Lincoln, YS and Guba, EG (1990) *Naturalistic Inquiry*. 7th edition. Newbury Park, CA: Sage.

Madden, R (2010) *Being Ethnographic: A Guide to the Theory and Practice of Ethnography*. London: Sage.

McDermid, F, Peters, K, Jackson, D and Daly, J (2014) Conducting qualitative research in the context of pre-existing peer and collegial relationships. *Nurse Researcher* 21(5): 28–33.

Mills, CW (1959) *The Sociological Imagination*. New York: Oxford University Press.

Moffat, A (2008) *The Reivers: The Story of the Border Reivers*. Edinburgh: Birlinn.

Monahan, T and Fisher, JA (2010) Benefits of 'observer effects': lessons from the field. *Qualitative Research* 10(3): 357–376.

Mykhalovskiy, E (1996) Reconsidering table talk: critical thoughts on the relationship between sociology, autobiography and self-indulgence. *Qualitative Sociology* 19(1): 131–151.

Pereira de Melo, L, Stofel, N, Gualda, D and Campos, E (2014) Nurses' experiences of ethnographic fieldwork. *Nurse Researcher* 22(1): 14–19.

Reinharz, S (Ed) (1997) *Reflexivity and Voice*. Thousand Oaks, CA: Sage.

Robertson, S (2006) Masculinity and reflexivity in health research with men. *Auto/biography* 14(1): 1–18.

Schensul, JJ and LeCompte, MD (2013) *Essential Ethnographic Methods: A Mixed Methods Approach*. 2nd edition. Lanham, MD: Alta Mira Press.

Simmons, M (2007) Insider ethnography: tinker, tailor, researcher or spy? *Nurse Researcher* 14(4): 7–17.

Stanley, L and Wise, S (1993) *Breaking Out Again: Feminist Ontology and Epistemology*. 2nd edition. London: Routledge.

Steibel, D, Caron, NA and Lopes, RS (2014) An observer's intense and challenging journey observing the short life of an extremely premature baby in neonatal intensive care. *Infant Observation* 17(3): 233–247.

Treyvaud, K (2014) Parent and family outcomes following very preterm or very low birth weight birth: a review. *Seminars in Fetal and Neonatal Medicine* 19(2): 131–135.

Turner, JH (2009) The sociology of emotions: basic theoretical arguments. *Emotion Review* 1(4): 340–354.

Walker, K (1997) Cutting edges: deconstructive inquiry and the mission of the border ethnographer. *Nursing Inquiry* 4(1): 3–13.

Weightman, AL, Morgan, HE, Shepherd, MA, Kitcher, H, Roberts, C and Dunstan, FD (2012) Social inequality and infant health in the UK: systematic review and meta-analyses. *BMJ Open* 2: e000964. DOI:10.1136/bmjopen-2012-000964

Wilson, VJ, McCormack, BG and Ives, G (2005) Understanding the workplace culture of a special care nursery. *Journal of Advanced Nursing* 50(1): 27–38.

9

EVALUATIVE ETHNOGRAPHY FOR MATERNAL AND CHILD NUTRITION INTERVENTIONS

Sera Young and Gretel H. Pelto

Introduction

This chapter is intended to provide an overview of evaluative ethnography in public health, with a special emphasis on maternal and child nutrition interventions. We define "evaluative ethnography" as qualitative research that is grounded in ethnographic techniques and theories, and that is undertaken to inform and improve the translational process from discovery-oriented research to implementation research. Evaluative ethnography of the social and political processes that lead to the policies that enables an intervention is also essential (Pelletier et al. 2012), but is outside the scope of what we consider here. Instead, our focus begins with the decision to establish an intervention.

The approaches we discuss are built on inputs and approaches drawn from a number of different fields, but they are fundamentally grounded in anthropology, which, together with nutritional sciences, is our professional disciplinary background. Consequently, our own work is particularly informed by anthropological methods and theories, and our envisioning of evaluative ethnography reflects this orientation.

Evaluative ethnography is most effective when approached with an analytic trifecta of strong theory, rigorous focused ethnographic methodologies, and a conceptualization or framework of study inputs and outputs known as the Program Impact Pathway. In this chapter, we discuss each of these tools, and illustrate their utility by drawing from a number of examples of applied work in maternal and child nutrition interventions from around the world.

Theoretically driven focused ethnography

The importance of a theoretical framework

The purpose of translational research in public health is to apply knowledge derived from discovery-oriented sciences, including epidemiology, to improve policies, programs and interventions. A fundamental challenge with translational research in public health is finding an appropriate balance between the demands for efficiency, economy, and other practical pressures, and the need for high levels of scientific rigor. Striking the correct balance is the perennial dilemma for applied research across a wide range of activities, including evaluative ethnography.

"Focused ethnography" is an approach we use to meet the challenges of balancing practical demands with the requirements of sound ethnography in interventions that are aimed at improving maternal and child nutrition. Generically, the idea of focused ethnography is simply that the research is focused relatively narrowly on research that is undertaken to support an intervention, and that it examines issues that affect the planning, conduct and evaluation of the intervention. This may be a program that is "free-standing" or embedded within other initiatives and addresses projects. To support decisions about what to include in the research focus, we think it is necessary to have those decisions grounded in a theoretically driven, empirically supported framework. The framework that an investigator chooses will depend on one's fundamental theoretical approach, and there is certainly no one correct theoretical foundation. The important requirement, we argue, is that the framework that guides the research be made explicit.

In our work we have found it useful to employ the "ecological model of food and nutrition." This model was first introduced into nutritional anthropology by Jerome, Kandel, and Pelto (1980), and we revised it in 2006 (Young et al. 2006; Young & Pelto 2012). It attempts to identify the multiple social and environmental factors that affect the nutrition of a population in a simple, but holistic, schematic. While aspects of society are not as easily compartmentalized as Figure 9.1 might imply, it is a heuristic tool that is useful for drawing attention to and organizing the complexities of the context of human nutrition. It aims to encompass biological and cultural aspects of nutrition through their linkage with diet.

The component labeled "physical environment" refers to the climate, soil characteristics, water resources, flora and fauna, land availability, pathogens, and other features that establish the conditions for food procurement and production. "Technology" includes the range of tools and techniques used for production, distribution, acquisition, storage, and preparation of all that is nutritionally valuable, including food and medicines. The "ideational environment" refers to cultural features, including beliefs about the role of food in well-being, cultural expectations related to health, definitions of food,

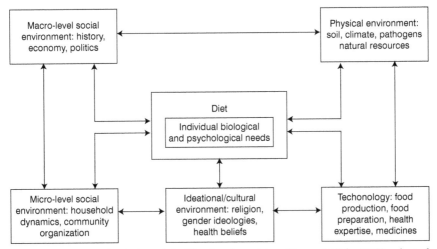

FIGURE 9.1   An ecological model of food and nutrition (Young & Pelto 2012; adapted from Jerome et al. 1980)

gender ideologies, food taboos, and religious influences on diet. The "macro-level social environment" refers to politics, economics, and history, while the "micro-level social environment" refers to household dynamics, community organization, and kinship structure. All of these affect the diet of an individual, which, in turn, influences and is influenced by biological characteristics.

In focused ethnography based on the cultural ecological framework, the selection of issues to examine is determined by first identifying potential issues and factors related to the intervention in each of the components of the framework. Some sectors will be much more important than others, but the starting point for the study design is to consider the potential role of each of them.

Focused ethnographic studies

Before turning to two examples of focused ethnography directed to infant and young child feeding, we provide some background about the development of the approach. Gove and Pelto coined the label "focused ethnographic studies" (FES) in the early 1990s (Gove & Pelto 1994) to emphasize three features of the methodology:

1   It is focused on a specific set of questions or issues for which data and insights are required, and which can be addressed within a relatively short period of research.
2   As discussed above, it is grounded in a strong theoretical framework.
3   It preserves the strengths of ethnographic techniques for data collection and analysis.

A "focused ethnographic study" is a mixed method approach, in which techniques are drawn from multiple disciplines and reflect different disciplinary approaches. The common ethnographic technique of open-ended questions, with exploratory probing, is a prominent technique, but the protocols also use survey research techniques (including 24 hour recalls of diet), as well as cognitive mapping and other techniques drawn from social psychology. As a descriptor of a research style, "ethnography" has come to be synonymous with qualitative research. However, small-scale survey research has historically been a part of ethnographic research (Bennett & Thais 1967) and ethnographic research techniques are not limited to the collection of data that can only be analyzed with qualitative methods. As Strauss observed in his influential book, *Qualitative Analysis for Social Scientists* (1987) the distinction between qualitative and quantitative approaches lies in how data are treated analytically, rather than in the types of data that are amassed to examine an issue.

Methodologically, focused ethnography typically relies heavily on interviewing respondents, using guiding questions that are intended to initiate a discussion about issues and areas of concern. These discussions are often captured with an audio recording, which facilitates narrative analysis. Thematic analysis is typically used to analyze the "text" created by the narratives.

When a study requires information on food intake, standard dietary intake procedures are used routinely and demographic and socio-economic information is collected with the types of questioning procedures that are used by many social science disciplines.

Some focused ethnography also makes use of cognitive mapping techniques. The basic techniques of cultural domain analysis were described by Weller and Romney (1988), and the use of formal ethnographic methods, including cognitive mapping techniques and their use in ethnographic research, was explicated by Pelto and Pelto (1978) and Bernard (2006). Applied anthropologists have made extensive use of cognitive mapping techniques as a methodological approach that facilitates the application of ethnographic techniques in rapid assessment/formative research (Gittelsohn et al. 1998; Schensul & LeCompte 2012). Two recent methodological texts in applied ethnography have outlined their utility and presented guidance on their execution (Borgatti & Halgin 2012; Pelto 2013). The types of data collection techniques used for cognitive mapping include free listing, pile sorting, rating and ranking.

In addition to cognitive mapping or cultural domain analysis, FES studies may also include social mapping, e.g. to identify sources of food acquisition. Structured observations and structured visual assessments in clinical settings have also been used. In a study protocol that included eliciting local names or "terms" for the signs of acute respiratory infections in children, videos of children displaying various manifestations of these signs were used (Gove & Pelto 1994).

Applying evaluative focused ethnography to understand the special challenges of infant feeding in the context of HIV

In the area of infant feeding in the context of HIV, we have used the ecological framework to identify domains pertinent to explore more fully with evaluative ethnography, as well as to make sense of data once it has been collected (Young & Tuthill 2015). Exclusive breastfeeding for 6 months, with continued breastfeeding until a minimum of 12 months of age, is recommended as the ideal way to feed HIV-exposed infants in low-resource settings (WHO 2010). Yet many women opt to introduce non-breastmilk foods far sooner, which increases the infant's risk of becoming HIV-infected and malnourished (Young et al. 2011).

From an outsider's perspective, the decisions to introduce non-breastmilk foods before 6 months or cease breastfeeding within the first year of life may appear to be counterproductive and difficult to understand. However, they often "make sense" in the contexts in which women are living. Applying the ecological framework helps us, the outsiders, to contextualize and understand how these behaviors can be seen as adaptive, from various players' points of view.

There is a growing literature on determinants of infant feeding in the context of HIV (Thairu et al. 2005; Tuthill et al. 2013; Bork et al. 2013); the following represent just a smattering of the many influences of infant feeding. Many women are receiving messages from their husbands, mother-in-laws, and neighbors that they are "starving" their baby by feeding him only breastmilk (micro-level social and ideational environments), and thus feel pressure to add other foods. Other women continue to hear outdated infant feeding messages, from previous national and international policies, that encouraged HIV-infected mothers to breastfeed for 3–4 months, followed by abrupt cessation of breastfeeding. Unfortunately these risky messages, which originated with a well-meaning public health community, continue to be conveyed to new mothers by some clinical staff as well as mothers who had previously been counseled on this message (technology and ideational environment). If a woman hasn't disclosed her status to those who care for the infant, she is often unwilling to explain to them her concerns about the important of exclusive breastfeeding (micro-level social environment). Other parents are worried about transmitting HIV to their infants, so would like to limit their infants' exposure to breastmilk completely (ideational environment). Further, in agricultural settings where women are expected to carry out heavy farm work (technological environment), this entails long hours in the fields away from their infant, making exclusive breastfeeding very difficult. This labor is sometimes made more difficult by the changing climate patterns in the past few years (physical environment). Other women feel that the stress of exclusive breastfeeding, together with her heavy workload, diet, and HIV status, is causing her milk to be insufficient to satisfy her baby (biological/psychological needs) and thus feel unable to exclusively breastfeed.

A research tool to use focused ethnography for interventions related to complementary feeding

The research protocol entitled *Focused Ethnographic Study (FES) for Infant and Young Child Feeding* is another example of focused ethnography in nutrition (available from: http://www.hftag.org/resource/1-fes-manual-v1-feb-2014-pdf/). This tool was developed under the auspices of the Global Alliance for Improved Nutrition (GAIN), who also supported its application in several sites (Pelto et al. 2013). The structure of the GAIN FES on infant and young children feeding was designed to encourage flexibility so that it could be easily modified to meet different research needs. The heart of the study consists of two sequentially applied protocols to understand household behaviors related to complementary feeding. The first protocol is for key informants (Phase I) and the second is for caregiver-respondents (Phase II). The protocol for key informants consists of seven modules, which include exploration of: i) foods for infants and young children; ii) food preparation and feeding practices; iii) sources of food acquisition and food expenditures; iv) types of problems faced by parents of infants and young children; v) food and nutrition problems of infants and young children; vi) health and food perceptions; and vii) perceptions about micronutrient supplements and fortification of infant foods.

For caregiver-respondents there are eight modules that are designed to provide data and insights about a range of issues related to household behaviors, including: i) demographic and SES characteristics; ii) a 24-hour recall for the index child; iii) food preparation and feeding behavior; iv) perceptions about value dimensions related to health and food; v) perceptions about factors that influence feeding of infants and young children; vi) perceptions about micronutrient supplements and fortification of infant foods; vii) estimated weekly food expenditure; and viii) food and feeding-related problems, challenges and solutions.

Over time, other protocols were added (or substituted) to examine issues of specific concern for the project the study was intended to support. For example, for a study in urban Ghana that sought to understand the potential for a commercial food, two additional protocols were created. One of these consisted of an examination of the local formal economic sector entrepreneurs, and the other involved the informal economic sector sellers (e.g. street vendors, people who sell from their home). In these protocols for studying local marketing characteristics, different modules were used to obtain data on inventory, selling strategies, sources of products, as well as on understanding sellers' views about their own motivations and plans, and perceptions about the population in which they operate. Elsewhere, for a series of studies in Kenya aimed at identifying potential agriculturally-related interventions, it was essential to examine food insecurity and the effects of seasonality on nutrition. Lastly, in the context of interventions to support home fortification of complementary foods, new modules have been developed to understand how families respond to and use new techniques for home food fortification to address nutritional deficiencies.

The Program Impact Pathway

In addition to strong theory and rigorous methods, the third basic concept on which evaluative ethnography rests is the idea of a "Program Impact Pathway," or PIP. The concept of PIP analyses has emerged in recent years as a means to convey an approach to the evaluation of health interventions based on the recognition that the effectiveness of interventions rest on a series of steps, each of which must be in place to ensure that the behavioral and biological endpoints are reached. The recognition of the complex pathways, in which there are facilitators and barriers to the flow of the intervention to its intended beneficiaries, is not new. Indeed, in the 1980s Rossi and colleagues introduced the concept of "program theory" in their influential work on principles and practice of evaluation (Rossi et al. 2004). In a theoretical paper in 1998, de Zoysa and colleagues examined the steps comparing interventions for vitamin A and prevention of HIV/AIDS.

The PIP is the pathway from an intervention input through programmatic delivery, and household and individual utilization, to its desired impact. Analysis of the process from input to impact is the basis for planning, training, monitoring (including supervision), and evaluation. One can conceptualize a nutrition intervention as a flow, in which the nutrient(s) and/or the information (e.g. behavior change communication (BCC) materials) enter into the delivery system and move through a sequence of steps, that lasts all the way until the deliverable is consumed or used by the intended beneficiary.

As inputs are placed into the stream, they can encounter problems, even in programs that have been very carefully planned. A bottleneck can be very serious, and bring an intervention to a complete halt. An obvious example is a break in a vaccine cold chain, in which the vaccine is no longer functional as a consequence of exposure to warmth. Everything that follows after the break may be fine, but the intervention itself is a failure. A partial blockage is much more common in nutrition interventions. This can take various forms, including blockages internal to the delivery system as well as blockages in the (household) utilization system.

Some common problems in programs in the delivery system that are formally reported in program reports or evaluations, or informally acknowledged by program administrative staff, reflect partial blockages. Examples of delivery system partial blockages include: i) nutritional supplements or medications not being routinely available at delivery points; ii) staff turnover leading to gaps in knowledge about management of the delivery process; iii) frontline workers not understanding the purpose or intent of the program; iv) frontline workers not being well trained on how to deliver the supplement or how to give instructions on its use; and v) frontline workers delivering incorrect information in the course of BCC activities.

At the household level, there are also a number of partial blockages, which are often identified in the "lessons learned" section of program reports or in evaluations. These include: i) the intervention failing to reach the households where the need was greatest; ii) for interventions that involve an intermediary to the beneficiary (e.g. infants and young children), caregivers not understanding how to give the supplement or how to prepare and feed the recommended foods; iii) other household members interfering with the actions the caregiver needed to carry out; and iv) caregivers trying the intervention, but failing to continue it. These examples, and many others like them, will be familiar to readers who work in programs.

The concept of the PIP as a tool for program monitoring and evaluation is gaining recognition in nutrition. In a project in Haiti designed to test a preventive versus a curative approach to reducing infant and young child malnutrition (Ruel et al. 2008), the PIP was used progressively and iteratively over the course of the study (Loechl et al. 2009; Menon et al. 2005). It provided the framework for designing both the "process evaluation" after the intervention was fully implemented, and the end-line evaluation to assess the success and comparative impact of the two different models. Other recent examples include one in Vietnam on the pathways by which the Alive and Thrive campaign impacted infant and young child feeding practices (Nguyen et al. 2014; Rawat et al. 2013).

The concept of PIP is also useful as an analytic tool for examining the performance of a class of interventions when one seeks to obtain a larger picture of common problems across a range of projects. To illustrate, Figure 9.2 presents the results of an evidence-based review that was undertaken to identify the role of maternal comprehension of growth charts in growth monitoring interventions. Roberfroid and colleagues (2007) used a theoretical model to examine the potential pathways through which partial blockages can occur in the delivery of a communication-based intervention.

Evaluative ethnography at three stages within the PIP: an overview

Full use of the PIP throughout the evaluative ethnography process depends on establishing a system of on-going information gathering, initially to provide a sound base for program planning, then to provide information about bottlenecks and feedback of the results to take corrective actions, and finally to use evaluation to make decisions about effectiveness.

Evaluative ethnography provides a means of obtaining critically important information at three key junctures in the PIP as described below. These junctures can also be thought of in relation to well-recognized stages of implementation

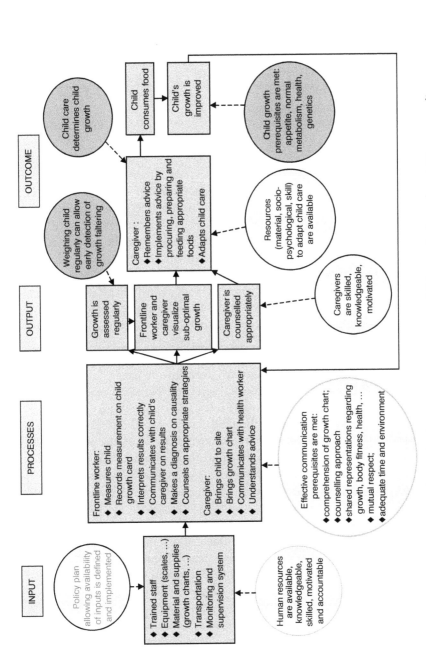

FIGURE 9.2 Basic components for a growth monitoring program to promote child growth through nutrition counseling

research in nutrition. There is no clear consensus about how best to label or refer to these stages, which is a cause of communication problems among investigators, agencies and donors. As the field of "implementation science in nutrition" matures, we can expect to see an emerging consensus about terminology. In the meantime, to avoid ambiguity and confusion, it is necessary for writers to provide their readers with their "operating definitions." In this chapter we use the following terminology: "formative research," "formative evaluation" and "impact evaluation."

Before the intervention: evaluative focused ethnography for formative research within the PIP

This label is widely used to refer to a great variety of short-term, focused research that is undertaken to obtain data for planning a specific intervention. Typically, formative research happens after a policy has been enacted and after a decision has made about which platform or platforms will be used to deliver the intervention. We use the term "platform" as defined by Ruel and Alderman (2013) to refer to the vehicle(s) through which an intervention will be delivered. The nature and focus of "formative research" varies widely. Typically, formative research studies employ qualitative research tools and techniques. This is sufficiently common that, for some audiences, the concepts of "formative research" and "qualitative research" are one and the same. We feel this is an unfortunate conflation of two very different concepts, one of which refers to a process in an implementation pathway ("formative research") and the other ("qualitative") to a general methodological approach. Not all formative research is exclusively qualitative; some formative research tools make use of techniques that involve quantitative analytic techniques.

A recent review of BCC, conducted with nutrition BCC practice professionals, revealed that formative research for designing the communication materials for BCC activities can be as short as two weeks or as long as two months (Pelto et al. 2015). Apart from its use in the design of specific messages and materials, formative research in nutrition may involve broad-based assessment of the delivery system and the utilization (beneficiary) "system." It may be used to identify gaps between best-practice recommendations and the current situation, and/or to identify facilitators and barriers in local cultural features that are likely to affect utilization. Another type of formative research, "Trials of Improved Practices" or TIPS (Dickin et al. 1997), engages with potential users of new products or new nutrition recommendations to find out if they are acceptable, or how they can to be adapted for local social and cultural conditions.

We note that another, related concept, "landscape analysis" is also widely employed in both public and private sector circles to refer to research that is conducted prior to initiating an intervention. In public health some "landscape analysis" is conducted prior to making a decision about which platforms to use to deliver the intervention. In other cases, a landscape analysis is conducted after a first phase of formative research to determine which platforms (including existing delivery mechanisms) are most appropriate or practical. Landscape analysis may be conducted as a "desk review," but it often involves fieldwork that resembles other formative research activities. Moreover, to make the terminology even more difficult to disentangle, some formative research is simply labeled "landscape analysis."

In the formative phase, ethnography may be used to identify the multiple features of the socio-cultural context that influence how a proposed intervention is likely to be received in a population. The ecological framework described above may be employed explicitly or implicitly to identify the sectors or domains that need to be examined. The framework calls attention to "who," i.e. "who" the key individuals in participants' lives are who could promote or prevent behaviors of interest, such as household members, clinic staff, or neighbors. "Who" can also include "gatekeepers" in institutions or communities, i.e. people who are critical to the planned activities taking place, such as hospital administrators or village chiefs. It also calls attention to "what," i.e. the commonly held knowledge about, understandings of, and familiarity with the behavior of interest. This can be used to identify, e.g. appropriate message content, training needs for study staff, and probes for behavioral recalls. Formative research is also concerned with understanding the "whys," i.e. the perceived needs, barriers, and promoters vis-à-vis the behavior of interest.

During the intervention: evaluative focused ethnography for formative evaluation/process evaluation/operations research

After the implementation of a program proceeds into full-scale operation, there comes a point at which another type of evaluative ethnography is called for. In recent years the acronym "M&E" (monitoring and evaluation) has become popular to refer to a range of data collection and analysis activities. Under the heading of "monitoring," the activities may involve routine data collection to ensure that supplies are flowing, beneficiaries are being contacted, accounting procedures are being respected, etc. However, these "mid-process" activities may also involve much more complex evaluations that are designed to examine what is actually happening in the delivery and utilization systems. Much like the initial formative research, this type of research seeks to identify new facilitators and barriers, to see "what is going right" and "what is going wrong" in the PIP.

The type of research that is conducted in an on-going program is often referred to as "process evaluation" or "operations research." Another term that is used less commonly but is perhaps the most descriptively appropriate, is "formative evaluation." The latter terminology draws attention to a critical feature of the research – its intended purpose. There is little point in investing in interim examination if the results of the study will not be used to inform the process and address issues that are responsible for partial blockages in the

PIP. Like initial "formative research," "formative evaluation" requires that a mechanism be in place to act on the insights that are delivered. Ethnographic work in both the "delivery" and "household utilization" systems, together with small-scale surveys, provides a basis for mid-course corrections.

After the intervention: evaluative focused ethnography for impact evaluation

The third time point in an intervention during which evaluative ethnography is useful is for evaluation of the impact. As the name implies, "impact evaluation" is undertaken to assess how successful an intervention has been in achieving its stated goals or purposes. When the intervention has been mounted as a pilot project or demonstration project, the purpose of impact evaluation is to determine whether it should be expanded ("scaled up") into a full, on-going program. When it is conducted in a program that is already at full scale, impact evaluation may be undertaken to determine whether the commitment to the program should be maintained or whether other means should be found to achieve the same end.

Impact evaluation of public health interventions is a well-developed field of scientific inquiry. It is primarily a quantitative discipline that employs what are now well-standardized procedures for sampling, data collection and management, and data analysis. At first glance, this type of research would appear to be inimical with ethnography. However, beginning in the 1980s, and developed under the leadership of Susan and Nevin Scrimshaw, the concept of Rapid Assessment Procedures (RAP) brought ethnography into nutrition and public health evaluation (Scrimshaw & Hurtado 1987; Scrimshaw & Gleason 1992).

At a general level, the types of questions that can be explored with ethnography for impact evaluation are similar to those of process evaluation: the participants' understanding of the purposes of the intervention; barriers and promoters to participation in the intervention; and the perceived benefits and dis-benefits to the nutritional, physical, mental and possibly spiritual well-being of the participant and others touched by her participation (infant, husband, neighbors, etc.). Although this is arguably some of the most valuable data, in that it permits evaluation of the entire experience of involvement with an intervention, formal use of ethnographic techniques for impact evaluation is not common. There are many reasons for this. Evaluation after a study can be logistically fraught—especially in programs or studies that have slower-than-anticipated recruitment, pushing study closure past deadlines, or in studies that go over budget, leaving no funds for analysis, or both.

Informal qualitative evaluations of interventions are actually quite common. In infant and young child feeding interventions, for example, the significant role of barriers in the intervention pathway are usually included in a "lessons learned" section devoted to identifying and discussing the nodes in the implementation pathway where failure to overcome barriers reduced effectiveness. However, data to inform these insights have generally not been collected or analyzed in rigorous, systematic ways. Moreover, "lessons learned" have not been systematically reviewed, and thus lose their potential power to contribute to a stronger theoretical framework for nutrition interventions.

Examples of evaluative focused ethnography for formative research

We will offer two examples to illustrate the utility of ethnography in formative work. The first comes from our work on pica among Mexican-born women living in the US, and the second from infant feeding practices among Kenyan women of mixed HIV status.

Preparing for an observational study of pica among Mexican-born women

Pica is the craving and subsequent consumption of non-food items. Earth (geophagy), raw starch (amylophagy), and large quantities of ice (pagophagy) are the most commonly craved items, but there are many other craved non-foods that vary by location (Young 2010). The causes and health consequences are not fully understood for a number of reasons, many of which can actually be attributed to lack of formative work (Young 2011). For example, clinicians and researchers often do not query about it, or when they do, they use judgmental language or inquire about items not commonly craved in that population.

It became clear to us that more information was needed about the prevalence of pica during pregnancy among minority populations in the United States, especially among Latinos. Because pica can be a stigmatized behavior, it was important to probe appropriately. Therefore, as a prelude to a large population-based survey, we conducted nine focus-group discussions with 76 women (23 in the United States, 53 in Mexico) (Lin et al. 2014).

Analysis of data from these focus-group discussions, including the transcripts as well as notes about participants' behavior and demeanor during the discussions, yielded a number of important insights that were then incorporated into the survey. First, the frequency with which participants reported personally engaging in pica (37 percent) or knowing others who had engaged in pica suggested that the survey would identify many with pica. Second, this formative research made it possible to create a list of specific substances to be queried about systematically. Some items were expected, but others including unripe mango and uncooked rice, were substances that had not previously been reported as items that women in this population crave. Further, it became clear that geophagic substances should be queried with a phrase like "sucked on" (*chupando*), rather than "consumed." Last, it was clear that women were conflicted over their behavior; women thought harm could come to the infant if cravings were not indulged, but that if they were indulged, the items craved could be harmful. Data from the survey are currently being analyzed.

Preparing for a cohort study of the effects of food insecurity among pregnant and lactating Kenyan women

A second example of focused evaluative ethnography in formative work comes from preparation for an observational cohort study in Nyanza province, Kenya. We have hypothesized that food insecurity can impact the health, nutritional status, and psychosocial well-being of both mothers and infants, and intend to quantitatively explore these pathways in a cohort of 360 pregnant women to be followed through at least nine months postpartum. However, prior to the commencement of survey data collection among the cohort, we wanted to be sure that we would be collecting data on all domains that were deemed relevant to food insecurity.

To that end, we engaged in a range of focused ethnographic activities prior to the start of the cohort (Dumas et al. 2015). These included semi-structured interviews with pregnant and lactating women of mixed HIV status ($n = 64$), their household members ($n = 10$), and clinic and program staff ($n = 9$). Our initial interview guides were informed by literature review, consultation with key informants, and our own experiences; these were then iteratively revised to reflect new issues that were uncovered during formative interviews.

Our efforts were rewarded, for a number of unforeseen topics germane to food insecurity were identified and could be incorporated into the cohort surveys. Some examples about unexpected perceived causes of food insecurity included artisanal mining practices, in which farmland is irreparably destroyed in the process of searching for gold, and female autonomy over resource allocation, i.e. who decided how money was spent. As for consequences, it became clear that the psychological burden of food insecurity was sometimes enormous, both in terms of the stress of experiencing hungry children, and also the shame of being perceived by community members as not having enough food. Questions about these experiences are thus also being incorporated into the cohort assessments.

Because we had expected that breastfeeding practices would be one of the most important domains to be impacted by food insecurity, we wanted to pay special attention to perceived relationships between infant feeding and food insecurity. We therefore conducted a small photo elicitation study with 14 women who had infants less than 12 months old. At the first of three photo elicitation study encounters meeting, participants were lent digital cameras and asked to take photos of all the people, places, and things that influenced the way they fed their infants. At the next visit, these photos became the organizing principle for the interview. The interviewer, a Kenyan medical anthropologist, probed participants about each of the photos she had taken, including what the contents of the frame were, why it was taken, and how it related to infant feeding. For the third and final activity, participants selected two of their most important photos and met together for a group discussion.

This exercise revealed intriguing relationships with food insecurity that suggested the need for further exploration. For example, it became clear that mothers placed a great deal of importance on being able to afford certain foods that were understood to promote her own milk production, especially cow's milk and cocoa powder. Further, the support of neighbors and friends for exclusive breastfeeding was experienced as an important determinant of a woman's ability to do so. Lastly, women's concerns about the consequences of their own diets on their breastmilk production were not unexpected. However, the repetition and urgency with which they conveyed concerns that their inadequate diets rendered them unable to exclusively breastfeed suggested that the biomedical community's understanding that a diet must be very low in calories for breastmilk production to be affected may need revisited.

Examples of evaluative focused ethnography for process evaluation

The Nutrisano study in Mexico

This case study illustrates the value of embedding ethnography within a larger study. The study was conducted by Bonvecchio and colleagues to improve the delivery of a fortified supplement (2007). This fortified supplement was promoted in communities using the informal term "papilla." The Mexican government had instituted a program that included providing poor families with a nutritional supplement, *Nutrisano*, which contained the vitamins and minerals that have been shown to be commonly deficient in Mexican children's diets. It was intended primarily to prevent malnutrition in infants and young children.

A previous randomized effectiveness evaluation of the program had found statistically significant effects on the nutritional status of children in households who participated in the program, but the magnitude of effect was less than expected, especially given the amount of supplement received by the households. An ethnographic exploration, which was conducted in two different regions of the country, revealed that a likely explanation for the attenuation of the expected impact was that household utilization behaviors with respect to porridge (*papilla*) were inadequate.

The formative research revealed that mothers typically mixed the *papilla* with a substantial amount of water to create a thin drink, rather than giving it as a thick pap or porridge. Also, a major reason for not giving it daily was that the ration was used up before the end of the month. The explanation for the shortfall was that mothers commonly prepared it more than once a day, gave it as a main meal instead of as a food supplement and gave it to other family members in addition to the target child. A baseline survey, with observation, confirmed the normative nature of these inappropriate behaviors.

The next step was to identify four appropriate behaviors and develop messages to promote them. These messages provided very specific instructions that could serve as guides for caregivers: (1) Prepare *papilla* with 4 tablespoons (SI) of the powder and 3 tablespoons (SI) of water; (2) Give *papilla* to your child every day; (3) Give *papilla* to your child between meals, specifically between breakfast and dinner (the *comida*, which is best translated as "dinner," is the main family meal, which usually is eaten in early or mid-afternoon); and (4) Give *papilla* only to target children.

After the messages were defined, a number of steps were undertaken to promote the new messages, including identifying additional channels to interact with families, in addition to health workers who were already involved in the delivery system for the messages. The team also developed a variety of new communication techniques. These techniques were implemented in two locations – a rural, non-Indigenous area, and an Indigenous area in the south of the country.

The next round of research was undertaken to assess the effectiveness of the new communication strategy to improve caregiving. It included the collection of survey data and focus-group discussions. An observational component provided an opportunity to examine mothers' behaviors and compare them to what they reported in the final survey. The results showed that messages 1, 2 and 3 were very successful, but many mothers did not accept message 4 and continued to give the *papilla* to other young children in the households. This was especially the case in the Indigenous area.

The qualitative results from the focus groups helped to interpret the survey results. In the Indigenous area, the cultural norms militated against singling out one child for special treatment. The mothers in the non-Indigenous area were also uncomfortable about not sharing something valuable with other children. The ethnographic component also provided insights for what to do about the problem of continued sharing. One mother suggested that households should be provided with a sufficient quantity of the supplement to enable mothers to give it to other young children. She said: "When you have more than one child and the three-year-old is the only one that receives *papilla*, she is the only one that eats it, so the others start to cry. I feel sorry for them because we cannot give them the *papilla*… then I see that there is a problem. For this reason I think all the children in the family should receive the *papilla*."

Process evaluation in a micronutrient supplement trial in Haiti

This example concerns a study designed to examine the feasibility and acceptability of distributing micronutrient powders as part of a food-assisted maternal and child health and nutrition program in rural Haiti. In this study, we developed a PIP analysis to identify critical points along the delivery and household utilization pathway and determine what data collection procedures to employ to be sure that the intervention was being implemented as planned.

Both quantitative and qualitative methods were employed, including focus group discussions (FGD) and individual interviews with program staff and with beneficiaries.

The transcripts of the discussions with program staff and with program participants were analyzed separately. These data were supplemented with the interviewer's field notes, which provided information on the participants, the context of the interviews, and the interviewer's own reflections about the interview.

An important finding from the interviews with staff was their experience of the increased workload the new intervention entailed. This was particularly the case for the frontline workers who functioned as "health promoters." For example, one health promoter said: "This is an enormous work increase; if one has 5 clubs [referring to the small social support gatherings that met routinely for BCC activities] one is obliged to talk about the supplement use in the 5 clubs. And in some clubs one is obliged to repeat the education several times so that everybody understands it. I think that this is an additional task."

While some staff members found the additional work to be burdensome, many of them also expressed the personal rewards they experienced, in spite of the additional work. As is often the case with the revelations that come from ethnography, the investigators had not anticipated what these would be. For example, one articulate frontline worker said: "But we have to say as well that we accept this increased workload because it is something related to health, and it makes our work more interesting because if the people come and take away something, this raises our reputation in their eyes" (Health promoter).

The discussions with caregivers provided insights into their experiences and indicated that these were generally positive. The following are illustrative:

> [The supplement distribution] is a very good thing. My child was weighed last month and weighed 12 kg. This month, his weight increased, this is because of the supplement. In addition, the child now eats very well.

> The supplement helps the child to develop. He gets iron. This is why I think that [the Sprinkles distribution] is a good thing.

> When my child had dark stools, I was worried, but now I know that this is nothing because before starting to distribute [the supplement] we were told that the child could have dark stools.

A benefit of ethnographic data, which is often overlooked in formative research-oriented discussions about the value of collecting qualitative data, is its role in supporting the validity of survey results. In the Haiti trial the household survey results were generally quite positive. They suggested that caregivers understood the value of the supplement and were using it correctly. But to what extent were these affirmations correct? Were the respondents simply telling the researchers what they thought we wanted to hear in order to keep the other benefits of the program? The breadth of knowledge the caregivers demonstrated in their discussions and the appropriateness of their motivations for using the supplements was reassuring. It suggested that the project had successfully engaged with women, and the survey answers reflected a larger cultural reality.

Examples of ethnography in impact evaluation

Evaluative ethnography can reveal the surprisingly multi-factorial nature of the impacts of maternal and child nutrition interventions. Here, we draw examples from two very different types of intervention studies.

The impacts of a breastmilk pasteurization intervention among HIV-infected Tanzanian women

Heat-treating breastmilk has been an infant feeding option recommended by the World Health Organization as a strategy to reduce vertical transmission since at least 2000 (WHO 2010; WHO/UNICEF/UNAIDS 2000). However, little was known about women's actual experiences with it. Therefore, we conducted the Makilika study, a home-based infant feeding counseling intervention in which breastmilk pasteurization was encouraged by peer counselors after 6 months of exclusive breastfeeding, to HIV-infected mothers with HIV-uninfected infants (Chantry et al. 2012). Mothers were then followed until their infants were 9 months old to understand behaviors and experiences with breastmilk pasteurization. While the study was on-going, we conducted 19 in-depth interviews with study participants and three FGDs with peer counselors. In May 2011, two years after the conclusion of the Makilika study, we conducted a fourth FGD with two study participants and two peer counselors, to further explore the impact of the study (Young et al. 2013).

The final focus group discussion suggested that the experiences with the Makilika study stayed with both staff and mothers, even two years after the study had concluded. Study participants and counselors alike were adamant that more women should have the opportunity to learn about breastmilk pasteurization. Indeed, two years after the conclusion of the study, peer counselors continued to receive inquiries for support with breastmilk pasteurization. They also reported describing the process to many of the thousands of women they saw in the clinic. The mothers were also very staunch in their willingness to recommend breastmilk pasteurization to other mothers, despite its perceived drawbacks. Part of this commitment to pasteurization came from mothers' own observations of the differences between the health and growth of their children who received breastmilk and those who had not. Lastly, the nurses were concerned to see evidence of reduced HIV transmission among women who pasteurized their breastmilk. This was not possible because Makilika was not powered to detect statistical differences in transmission. As anti-retroviral therapy becomes more and more available, the need for breastmilk pasteurization as a large-scale strategy for prevention of maternal to child transmission is likely to diminish. As such, a large clinical trial of breastmilk pasteurization is unlikely to ever be conducted.

The consequences of macronutrient supplementation among HIV-infected pregnant women

Although there have been a number of studies of macronutrient supplementation in the general population of pregnant women, little is known about the implementation or effects of macronutrient supplementation of HIV-infected pregnant women (Siegfried et al. 2012). The nutritional needs of HIV-infected pregnant women could be quite different from those of the general population for a variety of reasons: greater caloric needs, greater morbidity and food needed for medication adherence.

We therefore evaluated the acceptability and use of a peanut-based macronutrient supplement among HIV-infected pregnant Ugandan women in Tororo, Uganda (Young et al. 2014). This study was nested within a large prospective clinical trial in which pregnant women were randomized to investigate the effects of two different anti-retroviral regimens on malaria (NCT00993031, http://clinicaltrials.gov). At monthly study visits, women received a month's worth of peanut-based supplements to be consumed by her, and 5–7 kg of instant soy porridge for consumption by her family. We assessed use and impact in a number of ways, but for the purpose of this chapter, we will focus on the "exit interviews".

Exit interviews were conducted with all women who had at least 4 weeks of exposure to supplementation, and were within 2 weeks of delivery. It was valuable to be able to speak with women after their exposure to the supplement for some period of time as the final assessments had evolved for some of them. For example, 100 percent of participants rated all organoleptic characteristics as "liked" or "strongly liked" at the first assessment, and 92 percent reported liking it at the exit interview. The exit interview was also a time during which participants could reflect on the consequences of supplementation in their relationships both within and outside of the household, such as conflict caused by requests for sharing the supplement, theft, envy or stigma (if the supplement is associated with HIV). The supplements were well-received, had a range of positive impacts, some of which were unforeseen Based on these findings, larger studies to evaluate the physical and psychosocial consequences of lipid-based nutritional supplements during pregnancy among HIV-infected women are warranted.

Conclusion

In this chapter, we have sought to highlight the importance of evaluative ethnography in maternal and child nutrition interventions. We have also attempted to prepare the reader for engaging in evaluative ethnography, by outlining its three principles: strong theory, rigorous, focused ethnographic methodologies, and the PIP. And it is our intention that the various examples of applications of evaluative ethnography in maternal and child nutrition leave no doubt about its utility to that area. It is our hope that systematic ethnographic analyses will become standard in public health interventions.

References

Bennett, J.W. & Thais, G. 1967. Survey research and sociocultural anthropology. In C. Block (ed.) *Survey Research in the Social Sciences*. New York: Russell Sage Foundation.

Bernard, H. 2006. *Research Methods in Anthropology: Qualitative and Quantitative Approaches*, Oxford: Rowan Altamira.

Bonvecchio, A. et al. 2007. Maternal knowledge and use of a micronutrient supplement was improved with a programmatically feasible intervention in Mexico. *The Journal of Nutrition*, 137(2), pp. 440–446.

Borgatti, S.P. & Halgin, D.S. 2012. Elicitation techniques for cultural domain analysis. In J.J. Schensul & M.D. LeCompte (eds.) *Specialized Ethnographic Methods: A Mixed Methods Approach*. Lanham, MD: Altamira Press.

Bork, K. et al. 2013. Infant feeding modes and determinants among HIV-1-infected African Women in the Kesho Bora Study. *Journal of Acquired Immune Deficiency Syndromes*, 62(1), pp. 109–118.

Chantry, C.J. et al. 2012. Feasibility of using flash-heated breastmilk as an infant feeding option for HIV-exposed, uninfected infants after 6 months of age in urban Tanzania. *Journal of Acquired Immune Deficiency Syndromes*, 60(1), pp. 43–50.

de Zoysa, I., Habicht, J.P., Pelto, G. & Martines J. 1998. Research steps in the development and evaluation of public health interventions. *Bulletin of the World Health Organization*, 76(2), p. 127.

Dickin, K., Griffiths, M. & Piwoz, E. 1997. *Designing by Dialogue*. Washington, DC: Manoff Group & SARA/AED.

Dumas, S. et al. 2015. Perceived causes and consequences of food insecurity during pregnancy and lactation among Kenyan women of mixed HIV status. *The FASEB Journal* 29(1). http://www.fasebj.org/content/29/1_Supplement/585.2

Gittelsohn, J. et al. 1998. *Rapid Assessment Procedures (RAP)*, Boston, MA: International Nutrition Foundation.

Gove, S. & Pelto, G.H. 1994. Focused ethnographic studies in the WHO Programme for the Control of Acute Respiratory Infections. *Medical Anthropology*, 15(4), pp. 409–424.

Jerome, N., Kandel, R. & Pelto, G. 1980. An ecological approach to nutritional anthropology. In N. Jerome, R. Kangel, & G.H. Pelto (eds.) *Nutritional Anthropology: Contemporary Approaches to Diet and Culture*. Pleasantville, NY: Redgrave Publishing.

Lin, J.W. et al. 2014. Pica during pregnancy among Mexican-born women: a formative study. *Maternal & Child Nutrition*. http://www.ncbi.nlm.nih.gov/pubmed/24784797

Loechl, C.U. et al. 2009. Using programme theory to assess the feasibility of delivering micronutrient sprinkles through a food-assisted maternal and child health and nutrition programme in rural Haiti. *Maternal & Child Nutrition*, 5(1), pp. 33–48.

Menon, P. et al. 2005. From research to program design: use of formative research in Haiti to develop a behavior change communication program to prevent malnutrition. *Food and Nutrition Bulletin*, 26(2), pp. 241–242.

Nguyen, P.H. et al. 2014. Program impact pathway analysis of a social franchise model shows potential to improve infant and young child feeding practices in Vietnam. *The Journal of Nutrition*, 144(10), pp. 1627–1636.

Pelletier, D.L. et al. 2012. Nutrition agenda setting, policy formulation and implementation: lessons from the Mainstreaming Nutrition Initiative. *Health Policy Plan*, 27(1), pp. 19–31.

Pelto, G. H., Martin, S. L., Van Liere, M. & Fabrizio, C. S. 2015. The scope and practice of behaviour change communication to improve infant and young child feeding in low- and middle-income countries: results of a practitioner study in international development organizations. *Maternal & Child Nutrition*. http://www.ncbi.nlm.nih.gov/pubmed/25753402

Pelto, G.H. et al. 2013. The focused ethnographic study "assessing the behavioral and local market environment for improving the diets of infants and young children 6 to 23 months old" and its use in three countries. *Maternal & Child Nutrition*, 9 Suppl 1, pp. 35–46.

Pelto, P. & Pelto, G. 1978. *Anthropological Research: The Structure of Inquiry*, Cambridge: Cambridge University Press.

Pelto, P.J. 2013. *Applied Ethnography*, Walnut Creek, CA: Left Coast Press.

Rawat, R. et al. 2013. Learning how programs achieve their impact: embedding theory-driven process evaluation and other program learning mechanisms in alive & thrive. *Food and Nutrition Bulletin*, 34(3 Suppl), pp. S212–225.

Roberfroid, D., Pelto, G.H. & Kolsteren, P. 2007. Plot and see! Maternal comprehension of growth charts worldwide. *Tropical Medicine and International Health*, 12(9), pp. 1074–1086.

Rossi, P.H., Lipsey, M.W. & Freeman, H.E. 2004. *Evaluation: A Systematic Approach*, London: Sage Publications.

Ruel, M.T. et al. 2008. Age-based preventive targeting of food assistance and behaviour change and communication for reduction of childhood undernutrition in Haiti: a cluster randomised trial. *Lancet*, 371(9612), pp. 588–595.

Ruel, M.T., Alderman, H. & Maternal and Child Nutrition Study Group 2013. Nutrition-sensitive interventions and programmes: how can they help to accelerate progress in improving maternal and child nutrition? *Lancet*, 382(9891), pp. 536–551.

Schensul, J.J. & LeCompte, M.D. (eds) 2012. *Specialized Ethnographic Methods*, Lanham, MD: Altamira Press.

Scrimshaw, N. & Gleason, G. 1992. *Rapid Assessment Procedures: Qualitative Methodologies for Planning and Evaluation of Health Related Programmes*. Boston, MA: International Nutrition Foundation for Developing Countries

Scrimshaw, S.C.M. & Hurtado, E. 1987. *Rapid Assessment Procedures for Nutrition and Primary Health Care*, Berkeley, CA: University of California Press. Available at: http://www.popline.org/node/367421

Siegfried, N. et al. 2012. Micronutrient supplementation in pregnant women with HIV infection. *Cochrane Database of Systematic Reviews (Online)*. http://onlinelibrary.wiley.com/doi/10.1002/14651858.CD009755/abstract

Strauss, A.L. 1987. *Qualitative Analysis for Social Scientists*, Cambridge: Cambridge University Press.

Thairu, L.N. et al. 2005. Sociocultural influences on infant feeding decisions among HIV-infected women in rural Kwa-Zulu Natal, South Africa. *Maternal & Child Nutrition*, 1(1), pp. 2–10.

Tuthill, E., McGrath, J. & Young, S. 2013. Commonalities and differences in infant feeding attitudes and practices in the context of HIV in sub-Saharan Africa: a metasynthesis. *AIDS Care*, 26(2), pp. 214–225.

Weller, S.C. & Romney, A.K. 1988. *Systematic Data Collection*, London: SAGE.

WHO 2010. *Guidelines on HIV and Infant Feeding*, Geneva: World Health Organization.

WHO/UNICEF/UNAIDS 2000. *HIV and Infant Feeding Counseling: A Training Course – Participants' Manual*, Geneva: World Health Organization.

Young, S. 2011. *Craving Earth: Understanding Pica, the Urge to Eat Clay, Starch, Ice, and Chalk*, New York: Columbia University Press.

Young, S. et al. 2006. Core concepts in nutritional anthropology. In N. Temple et al. (eds) *Nutritional Health: Strategies for Disease Prevention*. Totowa, NJ: Humana Press, pp. 425–437

Young, S. et al. 2013. Barriers and promoters of home-based pasteurization of breastmilk among HIV-infected mothers in greater Dar es Salaam, Tanzania. *Breastfeeding Medicine*, 8(3), pp. 321–326.

Young, S.L. 2010. Pica in pregnancy: new ideas about an old condition. *Annual Review of Nutrition*, 30, pp. 403–422.

Young, S.L. & Pelto, G.H. 2012. Core concepts in nutritional anthropology. In N. Temple et al. (eds) *Nutritional Health: Strategies for Disease Prevention*. Totowa, NJ: Humana Press, pp. 523–537.

Young, S.L. & Tuthill, E. 2015. Ethnography as a tool for formative research and evaluation in public health nutrition: illustrations from the world of infant and young child feeding. In J. Brett & J. Chrzan (eds) *Research Methods for the Anthropological Study of Food and Nutrition*. New York: Berghahn Press.

Young, S.L. et al. 2011. Current knowledge and future research on infant feeding in the context of HIV: basic, clinical, behavioral, and programmatic perspectives. *Advances in Nutrition*, 2, pp. 225–243.

Young, S.L. et al. 2014. "I have remained strong because of that food": acceptability and use of lipid-based nutrient supplements among pregnant HIV-infected Ugandan women receiving combination antiretroviral therapy. *AIDS and Behavior*. http://www.ncbi.nlm.nih.gov/pubmed/25416075

10

CHALLENGES OF ORGANIZATIONAL ETHNOGRAPHY

Reflecting on methodological insights

Daniel Neyland

Introduction

It's 2am on October 16th, 2009, and I find myself driving at speed toward the local hospital, my wife no longer able to convince me that she is not in labour. We are rushed through to a delivery suite and within a few hours our son is born. We are left by the midwives to spend some time with our new baby, but something is not right. My wife feels worse now than she did during childbirth. Is this what's supposed to happen? I go off in search of a midwife and she returns with a medical team. My wife is taken to theatre for a routine procedure. Meantime the baby is left to lie on me as I slump in an armchair. Having no young relatives, this is the first time I have ever held a baby. As she leaves, the midwife says: 'Try not to fall asleep.' I have been up all night, but I try to give her a look which communicates (without words): 'I am too scared to fall asleep.'

It's now 6pm on October 2nd, 2012, and this morning my wife was due to give birth by caesarean section to our second son. However, due to lack of staff our appointment was cancelled. Now (right in the middle of eating our fish and chips) my wife announces she is in labour. I find myself driving at speed toward the hospital once again. When we arrive, there are no staff at the reception desk. I leave my wife sitting on a chair and try and find someone. I find no one. I return to find my wife on her hands and knees in the corridor. I return to the reception desk and find no one. I return to my wife, unsure what to do. I then spot a person in uniform (possibly a midwife?) and rush over to her. My wife is taken to theatre and our son is delivered.

Childbirth seems to effortlessly mix the normal and precarious, mundane and emotional. Sometimes short or prolonged moments of anxiety are combined with short or prolonged periods of happiness and these are combined with the banal exigencies of being processed through a mostly bureaucratic (in my case UK) healthcare setting. During research work I try and maintain as far as possible the following rule: 'If it's going well, enjoy it. If it's going badly, treat it ethnographically.' Up until now I have not had the chance to consider childbirth with such ethnographic scrutiny. However, having been invited by the editors to write some concluding remarks to this excellent collection, I now find myself in a position to do just that. What I will do first is try and draw together a brief history of organizational ethnography and highlight some of the implications that this history might have for working in healthcare settings. Second, I will try and set out some of the themes that I found most interesting and engaging from reading the chapters and focus on what seem to me the most pressing challenges in doing ethnographic work in maternal and child health settings. Third, I will conclude with what, for me, was a key insight of the chapters: a move from inter- or multi-disciplinary research to studying collective concerns.[1]

A brief history of organizational ethnography

In a general way, ethnography involves the observation of, and participation in, particular settings (such as local indigenous groups, management consultants, medical students and so on). This observation and participation aims to engage with questions of how a particular group operates, what it means to be a member of a particular group and how changes can affect that group. Although ethnography has been central to the development of various strands of scholarly thought, it has also always been entangled with practical matters. For example, the origins of ethnography in anthropology were closely tied to organizational endeavours – namely the management of Western European colonial engagements. Here anthropologists to some extent sought to bring the 'exotic' back 'home' (for an example, see Evans Pritchard's study of the Nuer, 1940) at the same time as offering a basis for colonial management. The entanglement of ethnography with an aim to manage and organize the settings under study has thus been of long-standing.

Throughout the twentieth century these ethnographic origins were taken in many directions through anthropology (for an augmentation of the 'exotic' through thick description, see Geertz, 1973), sociology (from the study of slums, see Whyte, 1955, through to youth culture, see Cohen, 1972), science and technology studies (see, for example, Latour and Woolgar, 1979) and the development of new avenues of exploration. Hence in the twenty-first century discussion of ethnography has found focus in considerations of the understanding and use of technology (see Miller and Slater on Trinidadians' use of the internet, 2000) and in questions of ethnography's ability to engage with messy, complex and chaotic organizational forms (Law, 2004) among many other areas.

These developments have continued ethnographic engagements with organizational settings. Anthropology continued to be closely involved in western colonial activities in the first half of the twentieth century. Indeed this involvement was crucial to the development of ethnography as a research method. For example, the early pioneering work of Malinowski (1929) and Radcliffe-Brown (1922) has been identified by many (see, for example, Burgess 1984) as providing the basis for the development of ethnographic fieldwork. Prior to these studies, many ethnographers had simply collected second-hand accounts of exotic lands from travellers returning to, for example, Britain (Urry, 1984) or had been involved in the development of questionnaire-type approaches to map out practices of colonial groups (Ellen, 1984). Malinowski advocated direct participation in the groups being studied and advocated using such participation as the central focus for developing an understanding of the group. The ethnographic principles of getting close to the group and spending a great deal of time in the group emerged at this time.

Baba (2005) suggests that the popular view that this colonial entanglement provides something of a blot on the history of ethnography, is a relatively recent reading of events and that early anthropology involved both practical and scholarly pursuits. She argues that "In the past, relationships between pragmatic and scholarly interests were fuzzier and more entangled than the received version would have us believe" (2005:206). Drawing on the work of Kuper (1983) she points out that forms of applied anthropology date from at least 1881: "when British anthropologists used it to advocate the potential utility of their emerging profession which did not yet have a firm constituency" (2005:206). Early ethnography combined practical and scholarly pursuits, but not in seamless ways. Often practical work (depending on funding and availability) was handed over to junior colleagues (often women), beginning a separation between (more esteemed) theory and (lower status) practice.

Histories of ethnography (such as Baba, 2005) suggest that the funding for such theoretical-practical work continued through the Second World War in line with endeavours to engage with colonial groups. Post-independence and the end of empire, such interest dwindled. Schwartzman (1993) argues that simultaneous to the decline in colonial, practical studies, anthropology moved into new and distinct settings, raising new practical questions for ethnography. The Hawthorne studies of the 1920s and 1930s involved ethnography moving in to the workplace. Schwartzman highlights how Lloyd Warner suggested "work groups could be studied as a type of small society" (1993:9). Although these studies were subsequently criticized for apparently representing the workers as less logical than their superiors, this research began to indicate that anthropological techniques, spending time in the setting, producing a detailed picture of the mundane and the ordinary, could have potential for studies 'at home' as much as in 'exotic' locations abroad. The practical approach taken by these ethnographers was emphasized by Lloyd Warner who went on to found a consulting firm, Social Research, Inc.

In recent years there has been something of a reinvigoration of questions of ethnographic utility for organizational settings. The Xerox Paolo-Alto Research Centre (PARC) employment of ethnographers has renewed questions of ethnographic research and the possibility of combining scholarly ethnographic research with practical and pragmatic considerations. Suchman (2000) has even asked if anthropology itself has now become a brand. But anthropology has not had an exclusive hold on the use of ethnography for social science research. While anthropology began through ethnographic engagements with 'exotic' tribes in far-flung places, sociological ethnography began with subject matter closer to home. These sociological beginnings also drew together ethnography as a scholarly pursuit with practical and pragmatic (in this case, political) questions. The Chicago School (for a discussion, see Fielding, 2001) used ethnography for the practical political purpose of enhancing knowledge of particular groups within inner-city slums who, they claimed, were poorly represented by statistical analyses which offered little information on who people were, what they did, how they organized their lives and what problems they faced. Ethnography was deployed here in order to get close to those who dwelt in the poorer areas of cities in order to make available insights into their lives which might provide some political leverage. The explicit political aim of the likes of Whyte (1955) and his study of the street-corner life of Boston slums, was one of adequate representation.

These studies were not designed to make available the obvious, or 'things we all know about' the particular group under study. Instead these studies made available detailed, insightful and often counter-intuitive pictures of, amongst other things, the complex organization of marijuana users (Becker, 1973) and fighting between rival gangs (Cohen, 1972). This counter-intuitive aspect of ethnographic research has been important in making available detailed analysis of the activities of particular groups which had been absent from media and legislative discourse.

A third and more recent focus for ethnographic development has been the field of management research. Sporadic calls have been made for the relevance of ethnography for addressing quite traditional concerns within organizational and management research. In for example, organizational behaviour (Bergman, 2003), strategy (Whittington, 2004) and accounting research (Dey, 2002), forms of ethnographic research have been utilized in order to address questions of 'culture', 'strategic practice' and 'change'. However, the separation between management research and anthropology is not clear-cut (see for example, Darrah, 1996; Rosen, 2000). Baba (1986) suggests that the origins of organizational behaviour lie in anthropological research such as the Hawthorne studies. It was in these studies that the grounds for in-depth, up-close studies of the everyday, routinized, informal activities of the workplace were established.

Czarniawska-Joerges (1992) traces the historical shifts which saw the fields of anthropology and management research move apart over time. She suggests that organizational-management research developed rapidly in the 1950s and 60s, moving away from anthropological ideas towards supposedly scientific notions being developed in much sociological research at the time (for example, sociological researchers were pushing the development of survey sampling techniques, statistical formulae, experimental designs and data processing). However, Bate (1997) argues that it may be time for reconciliation. Bate identifies moves being made in the UK and more prominently in the US to bring together anthropological and organizational behaviour concerns, highlighting the importance of getting close to subjects under study, making available routine aspects of organizational activity for analysis and studying 'history' and 'context'. Furthermore, although management and anthropological research has been separated in the past by anthropologists' study of the exotic and management researchers' focus on organizations 'at home' (Burack, 2002), this is no longer such a clear distinction with many anthropologists also studying the exotic at home.

In line with sociological ethnographies which sought to question 'what we all know about' particular groups through, for example, media reportage, Bate (1997) suggests that organizational ethnography has an important part to play in management research by demonstrating counter-intuitive aspects of organizational activity. Bate draws on examples such as Latour and Woolgar's (1979) study of laboratory scientists which suggested that objective, factual scientific method is far more complex and far less clear-cut than may be taken for granted. It is such counter-intuitive results, Bates argues, that offer ethnographic researchers the possibility of producing revelatory findings. Getting close to the organizational action is not just about telling the audience what they already know but also involves a refusal to take anything for granted. In the same way that anthropologists encountered exotic locations, tribes and customs, the organizational ethnographer can shift the everyday into the exotic, by carrying out detailed and close examination of their subject matter. In the same way that Chicago School sociologists made available rich and textured detail of life in the ghetto which (counter to media reporting at the time) demonstrated the level of organization of street-corner life, organizational ethnographers have the opportunity to scrutinize even the most apparently banal features of organizational activity to analyse what they suggest about the characteristics of the organization under study. For example, Weeks (2004) provides a detailed ethnographic analysis of organizational complaining, at once both an ignored and frequent feature of workplace settings. Through a thoroughly sceptical treatment of each aspect of organizational activity the ethnographer can get close to those everyday features of activity which hold the organization together. Van Maanen (1979) argues that the purpose of organizational ethnography is "to uncover and explicate the ways in which people in particular work settings come to understand, account for, take action, and otherwise manage their day-to-day situation" (1979:540).

This brief history of ethnography has suggested that ethnography in anthropology, sociology and management research has from its very beginnings involved a practical and pragmatic element, exploring the bases for organizational engagement. What might this mean for healthcare settings? In anthropological research we find attention paid to the continuing entanglement of doing ethnography and (attempts at) being useful. Pigg (2013) for example suggests that anthropological ethnographers continue to be pressurized to focus their research in ways that provide useful outputs for the organization under study, advocating instead: "a practice of patient ethnographic 'sitting' as a means of understanding, as a form of critical reflexivity, and as a diagnostic of the politics of relevance" (2013:127). Other ethnographic work in healthcare settings continues to push the counter-intuitive insights of ethnographic work by, for example, examining the complex ontological choreography of healthcare settings (Cussins, 1995), the ontological multiplicity of particular conditions (Mol, 2002) or the ways in which apparent healthcare futures establish accountable expectations for healthcare professionals in the here and now (Neyland and Coopmans, 2014). Being useful as an ethnographer in healthcare settings appears to continue many of the same themes I have briefly illustrated in the preceding history of ethnography: attempting to figure out a way to be useful for scholarly or more practical and pragmatic audiences; or figuring out a way of managing relations with 'audiences' who are not straightforwardly external to the research (but may in fact be participants in the research).

These kinds of issues should not come as a surprise. I have previously suggested (Neyland, 2008) that ethnographic research comes with a number of significant challenges. How to manage field relations with research subjects along with broader relations with the organization under study, the collection and analysis of data, timing, entry and exit from the field, questions of knowledge, ethics, research design and execution, seem as resonant in healthcare settings as they are anywhere else. What I found engaging across this collection was the number of different ways in which these challenges could be taken up, reported on and navigated. In the next section I will try to provide an account of what I thought were the main and most compelling themes of the chapters and the challenges they posed for doing ethnography in maternal and child health settings.

Chapters and challenges

I enjoyed the array of viewpoints and approaches organized among the chapters in this collection. I noted a number of challenges that were common across several chapters that were each approached differently by different sets of authors. I have arranged these challenges under five sub-headings here, but these chapters were sufficiently rich that they could have been re-arranged in a number of different ways.

Knowledge and ways of knowing

There has been a long-standing interest in ethnography with questions of knowledge and ways of knowing. These questions relate to both the forms of claim to knowledge made by ethnographers and the ethnographic study of knowledge practices within various settings (see for example Knorr Cetina,

1999). Ethnographic ways of knowing have typically (Neyland, 2008) been divided into, for example, forms of realist, narrative and reflexive ethnography. These each depict a different basis for knowing the world. Epistemologically they divide the world into different relations between, for example, the knowing subject and the known, and ontologically they treat the relation between the ethnographic text and the nature of the world in distinct ways. Hence realist ethnographies (see for example Radcliffe-Brown, 1922) tend to assume that the activities being observed exist independent of the study and could be gathered together as a more or less definitive representation of the group being studied. Realist approaches to knowledge are in many ways the most straightforward for questions of observation and representation. What is seen is taken (more or less) as a definitive version of what is going on. Narrative ethnographies (for example, Whyte, 1955) are often based around a notable informant whose views of 'what is going on' are taken as a valuable (but not the only possible) version of events. These narrative accounts of the field are often utilized to get close to a group who may not be easily accessed (for a discussion of alternative ethnographic styles, see van Maanen, 1988). The ethnographic account thus becomes one way of knowing among others without assuming that the nature of the world is itself easily accessible. Instead, more radical reflexive ethnographers suggest that the ethnographic 'reality' being studied is not independent of the ethnographers' work to produce an ethnographic text. Reflexive ethnography makes no claims for objectivity or knowledge neutrality, but rather seeks to emphasize its validity through reflexive subjectivity. The ethnographic text thus might constitute one (but not the only available) nature of the world.

It seems to me that these questions of knowledge and ways of knowing the world can become particularly clear when engaging with organizations. Organizational ways of knowing seem to stand in contrast to ethnographic ways of knowing on a regular basis. However, what the chapters in this book suggest is that although the aforementioned three-part list of ways of knowing (realist, narrative and reflexive) can provide a useful heuristic for engaging with knowing, the ethnographic practices of knowing, even in a broadly shared focus such as maternal and child health settings, can be varied and require consideration on their own terms. For example, Gammeltoft's approach suggested that collective ethnography involved different ways of producing knowledge and different combinations of knowing ethnographers (with insiders and outsiders to the community incorporated into the research team). In this way an ethnographic text moved beyond a single mode of knowing to a collective effort. As a contrast, OBoyle looked toward auto-ethnography as a basis for exploring professionalism. What got to count as adequate knowledge was a form of reflexivity, but one that might not just involve looking at oneself, but might also involve encouraging others within the profession to reflect on their actions. In place of a potentially problematic distinction between an ethnographic and organizational way of knowing, the distinction became a point for practical reflection. In a similar vein, Flacking and Dykes utilized reflexivity as a basis for exploring the ways in which the different backgrounds of each author constituted a distinct sense of the settings in which they researched.

Collective and auto-ethnography were not the only ways of knowing considered by the chapters. For Schmied, Burns and Dahlen, theory provided a means to frame their ways of knowing the field. Drawing on the work of Foucault provided a means to rework the ethnographic data and organizational implications of their study. However, alongside such theoretical concerns, the ordinary and mundane features of organizational activity also seemed to play a role in shaping ways of knowing. For Hugill, even the type of clothing worn in the setting altered the experience of doing research, the types of data collected and the expectations among other members of the research setting, including the research participants. Ways of knowing, for Hugill, were also re-oriented by familiarity with the settings in which the author had previously worked. When Young and Pelto described ethnography as a basis for supporting evaluation, it seems clear that as a way of knowing this stands quite distinct from conventional academic ethnographic relations of knowing. What I found most insightful about this range of approaches to questions of knowledge was that, as an outsider to maternal and child health, they applied to different (multiple settings, countries, procedures and practices) and the same things (maternal and child health).

Field relations and the handling of data

Closely related to the challenge of how to engage with knowledge and ways of knowing are questions related to the management of field relations and the data such relations produce. The time an ethnographer spends in the field almost inevitably means that they will strike up closer relations with research participants than, for example, a distant survey or even a brief interview. This close relationship is important for gaining in-depth, up-close views on what it is like to be a member of a particular group or organization. By participant observing the ethnographer becomes an effective member of the group. This membership can be illuminating for ethnographic research, providing insights into what status membership confers, how individuals shift from being non-members to members and what it means to cease membership. However, managing such relations can also be challenging. Ethnographers can establish rapport with one or a few key informants who provide much of the observational data for the research (Whyte, 1955), and can establish relations with gatekeepers who introduce the ethnographer and aid the ethnographer's move from location to location (Geertz, 1973). At the same time, the centrality of these figures to the data produced requires consideration. Furthermore, close field relations also engender relations of trust. Trust can be thought of as those close relations established between ethnographer and research subjects which lead to the mutual exchange of relevant information. Trust relations can involve work on the part of the ethnographer to establish that the research being carried out is rigorous, relevant and/or has some utility.

What I found in the chapters to this collection was a number of distinct ways in which authors positioned themselves among organizational members or managed such relations at a distance. These relations seemed to have direct consequences for the types of data collected and thus the study of the organization that resulted. For example, Brimdyr's study was informed by ethnomethodology and the orientation to get close to members' methods for making sense of the organizational setting. At the same time, and in line with other ethnomethodological studies of workplace activities, Brimdyr used video recordings as the basis for study. This research at a distance established a very particular basis for doing the research: that the members' methods for making sense of the setting could be studied through video and the ethnomethodologist's insights would not directly or immediately participate in those members' methods. Similarly, Taylor, Tully and Ball used video recordings as a basis for bringing data to attention.

Alternative approaches to field relations had different consequences for data collection and handling. For example, Gammeltoft approached the study from an anthropological approach, but also steered readers toward innovation through collective engagement with the field. Field relations thus multiplied. OBoyle's auto-ethnography was as much informed by a professional history as it was an opportunity to reflect on it, while also being infused with ideas of narrative as providing the basis for an informed and rigorous account of the field. In this way, the author's own history became an integral feature of field relations and the data it enabled. For some authors, field relations were not stable. In this way, although Hugill intended to carry out an observational study as a basis for collecting data, participation continued to be an inevitable feature of being in the setting.

However, 'field relations' could also become focused on the close management of organizational interactions, in that for Flacking and Dykes, for example, small rooms provided a difficult space in which to approach research (their presence in a small room seemed more like an assessment of research subjects) whereas larger spaces proved to be easier locations for navigating their research work and the sensitivities of participants. In a similar manner, Taylor, Tully and Ball looked to minimize the awkwardness of researcher presence by video recording night-time activity on the post-natal ward as a basis for removing the ethnographer from the setting. Field relations, the field site and the outcomes of the research were inseparable.

This diversity among field relations and types of data also continued into the handling of ethnographic data. Gammeltoft approached research accounts as matters to be treated with caution, providing opportunities to explore what was said in an account and what was partial or absented. Schmied, Burns and Dahlen explored the advantages of drawing together data by synthesizing multiple studies that they had completed. And in a similar manner, Flacking and Dykes argued for a comparative analysis across countries and settings and organizational scales. What I noted in the chapters was the rich array of insights achievable from following these field relation and data struggles between chapters; that what counts as good data or successful relationships in the field are never settled within a study, but can be usefully compared across studies.

Ethics

A third area that was noted among some authors was the issue of ethnographic ethics. Ethics have been a complex area for organizational ethnographers to navigate. From an academic perspective, ethnographers have tended to establish what the ethical requirements are in relation to their own academic institution and through local and national guidance. Historically, there have been three main approaches to ethics: ethics as rules which attempt to define in a relatively rigid manner the ethical direction of the research; ethics as guidelines which attempt to provide general principles which researchers should make relevant for each piece of research; and ethics as accomplishments through which researchers produce ethical outlines tailored to the setting for corroboration by academic peers, research funders and ethics committees. An alternative focus for ethical clearance has been the organizations under study. Access negotiations in relation to an organization can involve discussions of ethics, may require the ethnographer to demonstrate knowledge of the organization's ethical guidance, or alternatively the organization may wish to enter into a pre-research agreement on ethics. Such negotiations can be insightful in revealing concerns characteristic of particular organizations.

Despite the health-related subject matter of the chapters in this collection, ethics on the whole did not seem to have been treated as a significant challenge. Perhaps this is because doing research in healthcare settings comes with certain prefigured expectations and processes as to how ethics will be managed. Rather than act as a challenge to research, ethics becomes more like a standardized process. In the chapters, though, there was some diversity among the brief discussions of ethics which suggests that a single standard for ethically conducting research did not dominate studies. For example, Brimdyr suggested a formal approach to ethics with clear agreements in place, whereas OBoyle approached ethics as a matter of anticipatory self-regulation, attuned to the demands of auto-ethnography, and Flacking and Dykes suggested that ethical considerations resonated differently for the different national settings of their research. This suggests that ethics continue to be a challenge for the local management of ethnographic studies.

Findings

A fourth challenge that seems central to doing ethnographic work is the production of findings. This is challenging in a number of ways. First, there is the challenge of, in some instances, understanding and meeting the expectations of organizations in which the research is being carried out (I will say something more on being useful under the next sub-heading). Second, there can be a compression of time in organizational ethnography from thick description to quick description (Bate, 1997). Geertz (1973) developed the term thick description to describe a style of ethnography with rich story-telling of incidents in the field providing the backdrop for a developing understanding of the setting. To move to quick description suggests that the space between the initiation of research, its completion and the production of findings is compressed. This seems to threaten some of the principles of ethnographic research – that the researcher gets close to the members of the organization being studied, that time spent in the field enables the researcher to produce a detailed and in-depth picture of what is going on in the organization and that the findings emerge from the ethnographer's movement back and forth between previous observations and constantly emerging new observational materials (see Hammersley and Atkinson, 1995; Fetterman, 1989). Third, I mentioned in the brief history of ethnographic engagements which opened this chapter, that a long-standing quality of ethnographic research is to show something different, to not tell us what we already know about a setting, but to provoke and challenge our conventional ways of thinking. In producing organizational ethnographic findings, this poses the question: what can be said (and to whom) that retains the opportunity and ability to provoke?

Despite these apparent challenges involved in organizational ethnography, I found a number of ways in which authors had produced findings which upheld and extended the strengths of ethnographic research and even managed to provoke me to think in different ways. For example, OBoyle produced findings that were both insightful and provocative. OBoyle emphasized that what was important was the relation between a context of legislation and policy, and the actions of individuals (in particular midwives) who had to make decisions on professional standards and forms of care and the maintenance of their own professional status. OBoyle's own struggles with this continual movement between the policies and everyday practices and necessities of healthcare settings opened for me an opportunity to experience in detail the difficulties and consequences of those movements. I found this combination of relevant, but also provocative, findings quite apparent across the chapters. Hence, Gammeltoft suggested that decision making in regard to, for example, termination was a matter of attachment and detachment; intersecting theory with practice. Gammeltoft's distinction between heroic individual ethnographers and less heroic collectives could also act as a methodological provocation for ethnographers.

Other chapters looked to provoke in different ways. For example, Brimdyr suggested that moving others' expectations away from generalizable findings toward the importance of context-specific studies might be a challenge. In some senses, arguing for context-specificity might still prove a provocation for some. Schmied, Burns and Dahlen looked to Foucauldian notions of disciplinary power as a basis for questioning existing practices within maternity and child healthcare settings. In this way, the midwife was positioned as the expert in procedures and reporting but also in self-monitoring; internalizing the disciplinary gaze of the healthcare bureaucracy to such an extent that meeting targets might start to outweigh the needs of women in maternity settings. For Flacking and Dykes, being non-local provided a basis to treat everything as strange. In this way, being a non-native English speaker became an advantage in the UK part of their research as it continually prompted the question: what are these people talking about? And perhaps the basis for engagement (see next section) can itself be a provocation with, for example, Young and Pelto shifting the traditional academic virtues of ethnographic engagement toward impact evaluation. What I found across the chapters was not so much that the challenge of producing findings within organizational settings limited provocations or ways of doing research. Instead the organizational settings appeared to form the basis for innovation. I will explore this further in the next section.

Engagement with the organization

I noted in the opening to this chapter that ethnographers had on-going engagements with scholarly and practical activity. For example, from the initial development of ethnography in anthropological studies *of* colonial settings, we can also find the early development of ethnography *for* colonial management (Baba, 2005). Although some have suggested a division between scholarly and practical pursuits since its early development (Baba, 2005), ethnography continues to be engaged with forms of design (Hughes et al., 1992), marketing (de Waal Malefyt and Moeran, 2003) and organizational review (Schwartzman, 1993). While this ethnographic activity might, as Moeran (2005) suggests, mostly adhere to its origins in practising "long-term involvement with and study of the everyday lives, thoughts and practices of a particular collectivity of people" (2005:3), it has also on occasions become "a buzzword that covers virtually every kind of data collection available to market researchers, from telephone surveys to focus groups... [and] interviews" (2005:11). What we can note, then, is that ethnography in organizational settings both offers opportunities for innovation, but in innovating it also risks losing its methodological distinctiveness. However, we can also note a further challenge. Despite being provocative, and challenging audiences to think in different ways, and despite being innovative in method, it remains that ethnographies within organizational settings are often not just designed as a study of a setting but are expected to produce findings for that setting. Managing the challenge of on-going methodological innovation must on occasions sit alongside managing the challenge of saying something of use.

These twin challenges have been taken on in different ways by different authors. For some, an important feature of organizational ethnographic research is the progressive identification and accumulation, in the process of the research, of connections with participants and other potential 'users'. However, in line with explorations of "interactive social science" (Woolgar, 2000; Caswill and Shove, 2000) and engagement in research programmes incorporating novel forms of outreach (Woolgar, 2002a; 2002c), it seems that user relations cannot be taken for granted. The reflexivity which often forms a feature of the production of ethnography (Atkinson, 1990; 1992) can be extended here to considerations such as how and to what extent the researchers are themselves accountable for the value and utility of their research (Woolgar, 2002b; Neyland 2006). Careful consideration is required of the precise implications of utility in relation to organizational ethnography.

Assessments of utility form one feature of moves made to inaugurate a shift towards the marketability or customer orientation of research. As Du Gay and Salaman (1992) argue, there is hardly a public service organization in Britain "that has not in some way become permeated by the language of enterprise" (1992:622). This language of enterprise, however, is not a "vague, incalculable 'spirit,' the culture of enterprise is inscribed into a variety of mechanisms, such as application forms, recruitment 'auditions,' and communication groups" (1992:626). For Rappert (1997) one such mechanism can be found in university funding bodies' establishment of particular themes. These themes call for the "incorporation of users' needs," (1997:1) and suggest that "customer–contractor relations" (1997:2) are an important basis for research funding. This is ever more apparent in the UK with funders such as the ESRC expecting statements on the proposed 'impact' of research at the point when funding is applied for (rather than in a final project review) and 'impact' cases being made central to the Research Excellence Framework. These moves are positioned under broader motifs such as the "need to meet the challenges of international competitiveness and improve the quality of life" (Rappert, 1997:1). Gibbons (2000) ties this shift in research funding to the shift he identifies from Mode One to Mode Two research activity. Rather than setting research problems and solving them (Mode One), science and social science research is now more closely incorporated into the context of application for research and is produced via teams of mixed-skill researchers in close collaboration with users (Mode Two). In this sense organizational ethnography could be understood as shifting from study *of* the organization to combinations of study *of* and *for* the organization.

However, several social scientists (for example, Woolgar, 2000; Shove and Rip, 2000) warn against assumptions regarding the ease or comfort of interacting with practitioner audiences. Shove and Rip (2000) suggest "the over-reliance on an embodied notion of use and uncritical acceptance of associated pathways of influence is understandable but unnecessary... In short, the challenge is to understand better the process of use even if that means abandoning the comforting fairy-tale of the research user" (2000:175). This aligns with Woolgar's (2000) suggestion that "we should accept that users' needs rarely pre-exist the efforts and activities of producers to engage with them" (2000:169). These arguments contribute to a social science history of the difficulties of user interaction. For example, caution is advocated as to the "circumstances under which social science research enters the decision-making domain" (Weiss and Bucuvalas, 1980:248), with suggestions made that social science findings are prone to be misinterpreted, misunderstood or misused. Furthermore it is argued that social science is often "underutilised" (Wagner, Weiss, Wittrock and Wollman 1991:5), with findings on policy principles not used to their full extent. Warnings are also given against any assumptions that good social science will automatically be utilized. Thus Heller (1986) suggests that: "while only a few people would argue specifically against making use of existing social science knowledge, it should not be assumed too readily that a broad-based advocacy of more utilisation is either logical or practical" (1986:1).

The challenges posed to organizational ethnography in attempting to demonstrate its utility cut to the centre of the methodology employed. Concerns with, for example, ethnographic timescale and its mismatch with claims regarding the necessity of organizational speed (see, for example, Jeffrey and Troman, 2004) and organizational sensitivities regarding the provision of access for long periods to particular areas of organizational activity (see, for example, Harrington, 2003) are frequently cited as problematic features of ethnography's attempts at addressing practitioner audiences.

Despite these challenges, I noted in the chapters a number of ways of attempting to communicate useful insights and forms of ethnographic utility to organizations involved in the studies. For example, Brimdyr's study emphasized the importance of the first hour of a baby's life and the contact that it established between mother and baby. Further, Schmied, Burns and Dahlen suggested there might be an innovation gap in failing to bridge best practice between settings. Although these studies do not perhaps resolve all the preceding discussions of use and utility, they do point toward findings that organizations could seek to employ. Similarly, Flacking and Dykes suggest that their comparative study provided different findings in different locations, but also some common themes. For example, breastfeeding was a relational activity not a target to aim toward. And Taylor, Tully and Ball suggest that their study of night-time on the post-natal ward suggests a need for maternal support. Finally, Hugill argues that although the stress of preterm births for parents is acknowledged, the specific experiences of fathers requires closer attention.

This suggests a broad number of different insights of potential practical import. However, I suspect a number of the questions from the preceding discussion of utility still pertain. It might be that distinct expectations between organizations and researchers remain (Jeffrey and Troman, 2004), that a willingness to allow ethnographic research perhaps sets up particular expectations (Harrington, 2003), that users, use and usefulness do not straightforwardly precede research, but are entangled in the production of research (Woolgar, 2000; Shove and Rip, 2000), that without careful management research could be misused (Weiss and Bucuvalas, 1980) or under-utilized (Wagner, Weiss, Wittrock and Wollman 1991). Yet the chapters seem to tell a different story. This was not a story that denied these issues, but instead looked towards methodological innovation as a basis for exploring utility.

In this way, Brimdyr produced a study which was mostly designed to be productive for the organization studied: working through video as a basis for producing insights and following a model to provide steps toward sustainable change. OBoyle implied that through auto-ethnography, the professional practice of the researcher and the tasks of completing research could be drawn together. Taylor, Tully and Ball produced findings that were based on a study of the organization that might have useful implications for the organization, for example in suggesting that on occasions there might be insufficient staff on night-time post-natal wards. Young and Pelto suggested using a form of ethnography as a basis for impact evaluation and as a basis for supporting other methods of data collection such as surveys. The need for innovation seemed to me to indicate both the difficulties of doing organizational ethnography and the possibilities on offer.

On collective concerns

In conclusion, in place of drawing together the chapters and their rich insights (which have already been covered by the preceding description), I want to look at the idea of a collection in a bit more detail. What I have noticed, coming to maternal and child health as a relative outsider, is that the collection itself (rather than any particular chapter or individual insight) is of the greatest importance. It is the collection through which the value of the chapters is accomplished. In particular, the collection is where the challenges of disciplines and utility come together and are to an extent resolved.

I will say a few words first about disciplines before going on to say something about utility and why the collection offers a way forward. Drawing together a diverse collection of chapters such as those that precede this text, runs various kinds of risks. Different methods, different theories, different aims, different outcomes pose risks. These risks can be grouped together under the broad umbrella term of inter-, trans-, multi- or post-disciplinary research. I work in an area (Science and Technology Studies) which is often considered to be interdisciplinary, trans-disciplinary, multi-disciplinary or post-disciplinary. Like many others I come into contact with these risks on a regular basis. Much of my consideration of discipline and its risks feature in funding applications where I am explicitly called upon to demonstrate evidence of the breadth of conventional disciplines which will be incorporated into the promised research. Although I tend to use stock phrases in research proposals to demonstrate interdisciplinary activity, I have never greatly understood why I am called upon to do so or how these stock phrases might establish future commitments on which I will be assessed. Indeed I believe the stock phrases originate from a funding application written by a colleague (and perhaps he borrowed them from previous applications?). What remains clear is the expectation that the applications should be able to demonstrate this sought-after commodity. Although one could devote a research project to tracing the history of these interdisciplinary expectations in research proposals, that is beyond my scope here. Instead I would like to briefly explore four risks involved in doing interdisciplinary work and the general problem of assuming interdisciplinary research is inevitably an improvement upon disciplinary research.

First, interdisciplinary research often involves one approach simply taking on questions which have traditionally been the focus of another discipline. This involves a form of *empirical imperialism*. A problem with this approach is that the imperialist usually claims that they will address questions the original approach has found intractable by bringing in wonderful new insights from their own field – ignoring the possibility that the questions are likely to be as intractable, even given the fresh perspective, or ignoring the possibility that multiple disciplinary perspectives multiply problems.

Second, interdisciplinary research can involve one approach adopting the methods of another approach – a form of *methodological imperialism*. This often involves the imperialist attempting to export the method as a technique, leaving behind a great deal of methodological baggage. The result is the baggage is simply delayed in its arrival and generates problems at a later date.

Third, interdisciplinary research takes on the theoretical approaches of another area in order to address some of its own long-standing questions – a kind of *epistemological imperialism*. A frequent problem here is that the version of theory which gets carried across is hopelessly watered down in order to make it more palatable to the new audience.

Fourth, the notion of discipline for many scholars (e.g. Foucault) is tied into notions of punishment. For all the talk of inter/trans/post-disciplinary work, I still have the sense that inappropriate disciplinary transgressions are likely to be academically punished by peers who consider inter/trans/post work to be irrelevant to them (as it is 'outside' their discipline) or, worse, an impoverished version of acceptable work within the discipline.

I have the general suspicion that, at times, I have been guilty of all these forms of imperialism and attempted to gloss over problems with discipline. Perhaps this suggests that imperialism always appears reasonable from the perspective of the imperialist. The point of note is that discussions of interdisciplinary research can get hopelessly caught up with precisely what is meant by 'inter' and 'disciplinary' – do these terms denote forms of imperialism, compromise, engagement, development or something else? Are disciplines to be brought together to provoke, to fit seamlessly together or to inspire new ways forward? Is adherence to a discipline unnecessarily conservative? In the rush to proclaim our work as interdisciplinary (perhaps to secure funding), what is placed under threat? It seems to me that inter-, trans-, multi- and post-disciplinary terms risk losing both the history of a discipline (and these histories might provide valuable lessons) and the specific values of disciplines (in terms of both the 'value' of a disciplinary community and as a community with specific 'values' which can be drawn on in moments of engagement). The collection in this sense might be seen as a kind of risk, taking on the burdens of imperialism, disciplines and bland generic-ism.

However, I think this collection suggests a different way forward which eschews those risks and pursues a distinct way of approaching questions regarding the potential utility of organizational ethnography. As I mentioned in the preceding section of this chapter, explorations of interactive social science and the question of utility have suggested that research users rarely pre-exist researchers' attempts to constitute them. That is, researchers have to work hard to identify potentially relevant audiences and then convince audiences they should take part in research or dissemination because researchers have something of value to communicate. We should not assume that this operates in a comfortably generic interdisciplinary fashion. Instead, what the collection and its editors have done is build a range of specific insights, approaches, findings and provocations. The collection in this sense does not just build a text, but builds a world of relations into the collection, between researchers, approaches, organizations, provocation and their readers. A version of the world out there (readers, policies, histories) is brought to the research and hopefully proposed relations endure with organizations and readers who might find the content useful. However, for these relations to endure, explicit recognition needs to be paid to the characteristics of particular disciplines. For example, while anthropologists might work with conventions which suggest that attempts to demonstrate relevance can be made through drawing on ethnographic depth, those working in management research might instead be used to claims to relevance which draw on multiple case-studies' breadth. Similar differences might be identified between non-academic audiences. The assumption that breadth and depth and any other convention of proving can be comfortably drawn together or even switched in demonstrations of the value of interdisciplinary research, overlooks the values and commitments each discipline would seek to extol – attempts to bring disciplines together need to recognize this tension.

For me, this is where the key strength of this collection emerges. It is not a collection which seeks to merge or combine disciplines. It does not look to smooth out distinctions between approaches. It does not try to account for difference. In this way, the text builds a collective concern by gathering together multiple singularities rather than through mixing multi-disciplines into one generic approach. Alongside building a range of insights, approaches, findings and provocations, the collection involves a method (ethnography) and a topic (maternal and child health) which is simultaneously singular within chapters, but also importantly, multiple across chapters. For me it is this kind of multiplicity, which maintains disciplines (within chapters) while also offering disjuncture between approaches (across chapters), that builds an enduring collective concern.

Acknowledgement

This chapter was written as part of the MISTS project that received funding from the European Union Seventh Framework Programme [FP7/2007-2013] under grant agreement n° 313173.

Note

1 I have borrowed this term from an event organized by Christian Frankel, José Ossandón and Trine Pallesen, "Markets for Collective Concern?", Copenhagen Business School, 11 and 12 December, 2015.

References

Atkinson, P. (1990) *The Ethnographic Imagination: Textual Constructions of Reality*. London: Routledge.

Atkinson, P. (1992) *Understanding Ethnographic Texts,* London: Sage.

Baba, M. (1986) 'Business and industrial anthropology: an overview' *NAPA Bulletin 2*. Washington, DC: NAPA.

Baba, M. (2005) 'To the end of theory-practice "apartheid": encountering the world' EPIC Conference proceedings: 205–17, November, 13–15.

Bate, S. (1997) 'Whatever happened to organizational anthropology? A review of the field of organizational ethnography and anthropological studies' *Human Relations* 50(9): 1147–1176.

Becker, H. (1973) *Outsiders: Studies in the Sociology of Deviance*. London: Free Press.

Bergman, M. (2003) 'The broad and narrow in ethnography on organizations' *Forum Qualitative Social Research* 4(1): http://www.qualitative-research.net/fqs-texte/1-03/1-03tagung-bergman-e.pdf

Burack, T. (2002) 'Book review of "Turning Words, Spinning Worlds" by M. Rosen' *Journal of Business and Technical Communication*, April: 220–222.

Burgess, R. (1984) *In the Field: An Introduction to Field Research*. London: Routledge.

Caswill, P. and Shove, E. (eds) (2000) 'Interactive social science', special issue of *Science and Public Policy* 27(3).

Cohen, S. (1972) *Folk Devils and Moral Panics*. London: MacGibbon & Kee.

Cussins, C. (1995) 'Ontological choreography: agency through objectification in infertility clinics' *Social Studies of Science* 26: 575–610.

Czarniawska-Joerges, B. (1992) *Exploring Complex Organizations. A Cultural Perspective*. London: Sage.

Darrah, C. (1996) *Learning and Work: An Exploration in Industrial Ethnography*. New York: Garland Science.

de Waal Malefyt, T. and Moeran, B. (2003) (eds) *Advertising Cultures*. Oxford: Berg.

Dey, C.R. (2002) 'Methodological issues: the use of critical ethnography as an active research methodology' *Accounting, Auditing and Accountability Journal* 15(1): 106–121.

Du Gay, P. and Salaman, G. (1992) 'The cult(ure) of the customer' *Journal of Management Studies* 29(5): 615–633.

Ellen, R. (ed.) (1984) *Ethnographic Research: A Guide to General Conduct*. London: Academic Press.

Evans Pritchard, E. (1940) *The Nuer: A Description of the Modes of Livelihood and Political Institutions of a Nilotic People*. Oxford: Clarendon Press

Fetterman, D. (1989) *Ethnography Step by Step*. London: Sage.

Fielding, N. (2001) 'Ethnography' in Gilbert, N. (ed.) *Researching Social Life* (2nd edition). London: Sage.

Geertz, C. (1973) *The Interpretation of Cultures*. New York: Basic Books.

Gibbons, M. (2000) 'Mode 2 society and the emergence of context sensitive science' special issue on interactive social science, *Science and Public Policy, Journal of the International Science Policy Foundation* 27(3): 159–163.

Hammersley, M. and Atkinson, P. (1995) *Ethnography: Principles in Practice* (2nd edition). London: Routledge.

Harrington, B. (2003) 'The social psychology of access in ethnographic research' *Journal of Contemporary Ethnography* 32(5): 592–625.

Heller, F. (1986) 'Introduction' in Heller, F. (ed.) *The Use and Abuse of Social Science*. London: Sage.

Hughes, J., Randall, D. and Shapiro, D. (1992) 'Faltering from ethnography to design' *Proceeds of CSCW.* Toronto: ACM.

Jeffrey, B. and Troman, J. (2004) 'Time for ethnography' *British Educational Research Journal* 30(4): 535–548.

Knorr Cetina, K. (1999) *Epistemic Cultures. How the Sciences Make Knowledge*. Cambridge, MA: Harvard University Press.

Kuper, A. (1983) *Anthropology and Anthropologists: The Modern British School*. London: Routledge and Kegan Paul.

Latour, B. and Woolgar, S. (1979) *Laboratory Life: The Construction of Scientific Facts*. Princeton, NJ: Princeton University Press.

Law, J. (2004) *After Method: Mess in Social Science Research*. London: Routledge.

Malinowski, B. (1929) *The Sexual Life of Savages in Western Melanesia*. New York: Harcourt Brace and World.

Miller, D. and Slater, D. (2000) *The Internet: An Ethnographic Approach*. Oxford: Berg.

Moeran, B. (2005) *The Business of Ethnography – Strategic Exchanges, People and Organizations*. Oxford: Berg.

Mol, A. (2002) *The Body Multiple: Ontology in Medical Practice*. Durham, NC: Duke University Press.

Neyland, D. (2006) *Privacy, Surveillance and Public Trust*. London: Palgrave-Macmillan.

Neyland, D. (2008) *Organizational Ethnography*. London: Sage.

Neyland, D. and Coopmans, C. (2014) 'Visual accountability' *Sociological Review* 62(1): 1–23.

Pigg, S. (2013) 'On sitting and doing: ethnography as action in global health' *Social Science and Medicine* 99: 127–134.

Radcliffe-Brown, A. (1922) *The Andaman Islanders: A Study in Social Anthropology* Cambridge: Cambridge University Press.

Rappert, B. (1997) 'Users and social science research: policy, problems and possibilities' *Sociological Research On-Line* 2(3): http://www.socresonline.org.uk/socresonline/2/3/10.html

Rosen, M. (2000) *Turning Words, Spinning Worlds: Chapters in Organizational Ethnography*. London: Routledge.

Schwartzman, H. (1993) *Ethnography in Organizations*. London: Sage.

Shove, E. and Rip, A. (2000) 'Symbolic users – users and unicorns: a diagnosis of mythical beasts in interactive science', special issue on interactive social science, *Science and Public Policy, Journal of the International Science Policy Foundation* 27(3):175–182.

Suchman, L. (2000) 'Anthropology as "brand": reflections on corporate anthropology', paper given at the American Anthropological Association annual meeting, San Francisco, November 15.

Urry, J. (1984) 'A history of field methods' in Ellen, R. (ed.) *Ethnographic Research: A Guide to General Conduct*. London: Academic Press.

Van Maanen, J. (1979) 'The fact of fiction in organizational ethnography' *Administrative Science Quarterly* 24(4): 539–550.

Van Maanen, J. (1988) *Tales of the Field: On Writing Ethnography*. Chicago, IL: University of Chicago Press.

Wagner, P., Weiss, C., Wittrock, B. and Wollman, H. (1991) 'The policy orientation: legitimacy and promise' in Wagner, P., Weiss, C., Wittrock, B. and Wollman, H. (eds) *Social Sciences and Modern States: National Experiences and Theoretical Crossroads*. Cambridge: Cambridge University Press.

Weeks, J. (2004) *Unpopular Culture: The Ritual of Complaint in a British Bank*. Chicago, IL: University of Chicago Press.

Weiss, C. and Bucuvalas, M. (1980) *Social Science Research and Decision Making*. New York: Columbia University Press.

Whittington, R. (2004) 'Strategy after modernism: recovering practice' *European Management Review* 1(1): 62–68.

Whyte, W. (1955) *Street Corner Society* (2nd edition). Chicago, IL: University of Chicago Press.

Woolgar, S. (2000) 'Social basis of interactive social science', special issue on interactive social science. *Science and Public Policy, Journal of the International Science Policy Foundation* 27(3): 165–173.

Woolgar, S. (2002a) *Virtual Society? – the social science of electronic technologies*, ESRC End of Programme Report, University of Oxford.

Woolgar, S. (2002b) 'The boundaries of accountability: a technographic approach', paper presented to EASST Conference, University of York, August, 2.

Woolgar, S. (ed.) (2002c) *Virtual Society? Technology, Cyberbole, Reality*. Oxford: Oxford University Press.

INDEX

Bold page numbers indicate figures, *italic* numbers indicate tables